2584

WE870

CHASSAING,V.
Arthroscopy of the knee

Arthroscopy of the Knee

Vincent Chassaing and **Jacques Parier**

Foreword by **M. Lemaire**

Translated and edited by
Reginald Elson FRCS

Consultant Orthopaedic Surgeon
Northern General Hospital, Sheffield, UK

MARTIN DUNITZ

© **V. Chassaing** and **J. Parier 1986**

© **Martin Dunitz Ltd**
English Language edition 1988

Published by Masson, 120 bd Saint-Germain,
75280 Paris, Cedex 06

First published in the United Kingdom in 1988
by Martin Dunitz Ltd, 154 Camden High Street, London NW1 0NE

British Library Cataloguing in Publication Data

Chassaing, V.
   Arthroscopy of the knee.
   1. Knee—Surgery 2. Arthroscopy
   I. Title II. Parier, J. III. Arthroscopie
   du genou. *English*
   617'.582059   RD561

   ISBN 0-948269-23-5

Photoset by Scribe Design, Gillingham, Kent

Printed by Toppan Printing Company (S) Pte Ltd, Singapore

Contents

Editor's preface

It has been a pleasure to prepare an English text for this little book. I regard it as a simple and practical account of basic arthroscopic technique which will provide the ordinary orthopaedic surgeon with sufficient guidance to pursue a relatively new method of management. This is achieved concisely by word and illustration. I have tried to preserve some flavour of the French text. As always, I am grateful to my secretary, Mrs Valerie Barclay.

R.E.

Foreword

Fifteen years ago a young pupil of my friend Florian Delbarre showed me an arthroscope which she had brought from Japan. She had assisted the first masters of arthroscopy with meniscal resection, a procedure which was still completely unknown in France. At that time, I thought that the problems of sterilization of the apparatus imposed too great a risk of infection and that this outweighed the advantages. The young lady, however, a rheumatologist, had perceived the potential of the method and she developed a progressive interest in arthroscopy, accumulating all that was available from Japanese and American experience. It became apparent that sterilization of the instruments had become reliable and that, provided certain rules were obeyed, the risk of infection was negligible. Also, it seemed that both diagnostic and operative arthroscopy was without any apparent major disadvantages once the risk of infection had been excluded. Unfortunately, particularly in France, the popularity of the technique outstripped the publication of reports from the more respected specialists, who had had little time to report their techniques, experience, and their appreciations of all the possibilities as well as of the limitations. No really authoritative account was available.

Vincent Chassaing has taken on the difficult task of filling this void. In his book, he presents his views based on wide experience. He approaches the surgical aspects with great precision. In the same spirit, Jacques Parier and Henri Dorfmann have contributed chapters relevant to trauma and rheumatology. The text is embellished with diagrams and drawings by Denis Poylo. These allow easy comprehension for doctors who may have forgotten anatomical details.

In all, this book encompasses a general consideration of arthroscopy, its expected developments, its possibilities and its limits both from diagnostic and operative aspects.

The diagnostic potential for arthroscopy is enormous. It offers precise information as to the state of the synovium and of the articular cartilage; whereas information before its development was gross and very approximate. In earlier times, only major lesions at an already irreversible stage could be detected. They were then beyond the stage when conservative management would suffice, since this depends upon the early detection of minor lesions, associated with a clear understanding of aetiological factors. Rheumatology generally has been modified by the arrival of arthroscopy and the information yielded through closed biopsy. Lesions can be photographed and surveyed objectively, and the efficacy of various treatments can be appreciated exactly and followed progressively. There is, of course, a disadvantage in that diagnostic arthroscopy under general anaesthesia may be repeated excessively. However, I suspect that improvements in instrumentation, miniaturization, and perhaps the utilization of flexible devices will gradually reduce the need for general anaesthesia in a significant number of cases. Arthroscopy will then become a relatively innocuous investigation while necessitating a very rigorous aseptic ritual.

With regard to the place of arthroscopy in the diagnosis of traumatic lesions in the knee, it is probable that for menisco–ligamentous injuries, its place will become progressively less significant. Ligamentous lesions are diagnosed essentially on clinical findings; the majority of meniscal lesions can be recognized by good quality arthrography. The latter is a much less invasive procedure and provides adequate information. Further, other techniques may become available, such as magnetic resonance imaging: I believe that this will undoubtedly become the next major diagnostic development armamentarium.

Procedures like arthroscopy, which allow objective documentation and photography, are invaluable. Objective recording avoids the variation in interpretation which can occur between individual clinicians.

The range of arthroscopic surgical possibilities now available requires careful appraisal. It is indisputable that for two purposes it is ideal. Firstly, we have known for a long time that meniscal resection should be as limited as possible in order to preserve the protection of the articular cartilage; arthroscopy had made minimal resection easy and is now commonly performed, whereas by conventional surgery this was often difficult to achieve. Secondly, the remarkable instrumentation now available allows smoothing of irregularities of the articular surface and enables greater preservation. Other operations like the removal of foreign bodies from the knee joint, resection of synovial fringes and of the pathological folds, have also been made possible by arthroscopy. In ligament surgery, the attachment of the upper end of the anterior cruciate ligament has become feasible.

However, in my opinion, arthroscopic surgery presents a real danger. It is very tempting to resect a meniscus where the lesion of the meniscus has not been the only thing wrong with the knee, but has, for example, been associated with a rupture of the anterior cruciate ligament. The alleviation of symptoms achieved by treatment of the meniscal lesion alone may be immediate and impressive, but to allow the patient to return to sport without having done something to stabilize the knee takes us back to concepts of twenty-five years ago, when it was thought that anterior cruciate instability could be compensated by simple muscular re-education. Gradually we have come to understand the natural evolution and progression of instabilities of the knee and their aggravation by sporting activity. We know that such continuance will lead to progressive damage and to a severe arthrosis.

In summary, I believe that arthroscopy will progress in two main directions: diagnostic measures will be simpler and the examination will become relatively trivial while, on the operative side, arthroscopic surgery will often become combined with open surgery.

Whatever the ultimate development in arthroscopic technique, this new book will have achieved its aim in bringing us up to date with all aspects of the subject.

M.L.

Introduction

Physicians and surgeons have sought means to explore the inside of body cavities since the beginning of the nineteenth century. Early attempts began in Europe using progressively more sophisticated instruments for the examination of the bladder, the vagina, the lower bowel and the pharynx.

It was in 1918 that the first attempts at arthroscopy were conducted in Tokyo by Kenji Takagi using a system which did not incorporate lenses, aimed at investigating the early diagnosis of tuberculosis—a serious problem in Japan at that time.

At the same time Eugene Bircher was carrying out similar studies in Switzerland. Work spread and it was Kreuscher (1925) who stimulated particular interest in arthroscopy by the diagnosis of meniscal lesions. A little later, in New York, Burman (1931–1935) made other important contributions. Development continued with publications of work by Sommer (1937) Vaubel (1938) Wicker (1939) and in France, Hurter (1955).

In Japan, Watanabe (1957), a pupil of Takagi, published an extensive and beautifully illustrated work recording his personal experience.

From 1960 onwards, striking progress has been possible largely by the development of the Arthroscope No. 21 by Watanabe. This instrument allowed direct and lateral vision by the use of two types of telescope, both of small size. Irrigation with physiological solution allowed clear vision and a means of cooling the system. Photographic recording became possible. Shortly afterwards, in 1962, Watanabe performed the first partial meniscectomies; the second edition of his atlas of arthroscopy was published in 1969 in association with Takeda and Ikeuchi, again illustrated in colour.

Thereafter, it is impossible to enumerate all contributors, but mention should be made of Jackson, who studied techniques in Japan and introduced them in Canada and then performed the first removal of a bucket handle by arthroscopy; O'Connor developed the first operative arthroscope and in most countries there have been special promotors of arthroscopic technique: Gillquist in Sweden, Dandy in Great Britain, Johnson in the United States. In France, it was Dorfmann who first exploited operative arthroscopy in 1970. In 1975, the International Arthroscopy Association was founded under its first President, Watanabe.

The success of arthroscopy can be attributed to a number of factors, such as the technical improvements in the instruments (especially the lens systems), the introduction of cold light sources, increasing miniaturization of the operative instruments, and the use of video recording. Also, arthroscopic techniques have modified considerably; at first, observation was purely passive, but, with the introduction of the arthroscopy hook through a second port, the reliability of diagnosis improved enormously. Subsequently, various instruments have opened up new possibilities in arthroscopic operative treatment of lesions of the meniscus, the articular surface, the synovium, and in the removal of loose bodies.

The massive expansion in arthroscopic technique would not have occurred unless the numbers of patients had warranted this. Many disciplines became concerned and, while the needs of orthopaedic surgery have predominated, these others have become integrated: in rheumatology, arthroscopy has become important for both investigation and treatment, while in sports medicine, the ability of early return to athletic pursuits has been a particular advantage. Radiologists need to know the results of an arthroscopy in relation to their own investigations; physiotherapists and physical medicine specialists have been able to increase their understanding of joint function.

Our personal interest in arthroscopy has been influenced by many other workers to whom we are indebted and by whom we have become increasingly stimulated. We recognize freely that this book reflects the views of various schools, all of whom have contributed to our experience and current techniques. As a result of our own difficulties and concepts and solutions, we hope that the reader will increase his understanding of the knee and the practice of arthroscopy. The illustrative photographs and diagrams will contribute to precision and clarity.

It is our pleasure to thank Pierre Bories and Denis Poylo for the monochrome photographs and Jean-Paul Ceccaldi, Frederic Deltour and Chahla Miremad for the radiographs.

All photographs and diagrams relate to a right knee in order to aid comparison throughout the book.

1

Apparatus

The choice of apparatus is fundamental in arthroscopy since it is costly and any error will prove expensive. Selection is difficult because among so many authorities each will have developed certain preferences in various aspects of technique. Successive improvements also complicate the matter of selection at any one time.

Rather than detail an exhaustive list of available equipment, in this chapter we shall concentrate on the instruments to which we have become accustomed, while indicating the criteria that have guided us in our choice.

1. Arthroscope

The arthroscope (Fig. 1.1) transmits an image by means of a system of lenses while, at the same time, it conducts a source of light through a fibre-optic cable.

The direction of vision (Fig. 1.2) may be in the same axis as the arthroscope or it may be directed obliquely at 30° or 70°.

The 30° oblique telescope is the most frequently used and it permits an excellent exploration. Its obliquity enables the field of view to be increased if the arthroscope is rotated (Fig. 1.3).

The depth of field afforded by the optical system is particularly important. It allows vision of structures very close to the end of the arthroscope, and magnification increases rapidly as the object is approached by the end of the telescope (Fig. 1.4), a factor which is very important in the interpretation of the structure examined.

Currently, we use the 4 mm diam. Storz telescope in a 5 mm sheath fitted with two taps. The space between the trocar and the telescope is used for irrigation, either in or out of the joint, bearing in mind that the small size does

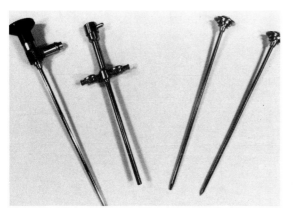
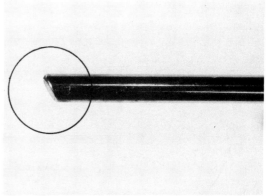

Figure 1.1. *Storz arthroscope. Sheath with two taps, and sharp and blunt trocars.*

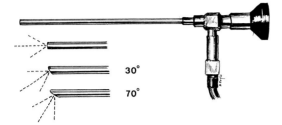

Figure 1.2. *Different angles of vision allowed with the telescopes.*

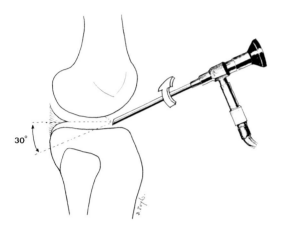

Figure 1.3. *The 30° oblique telescope is the most frequently used. It is necessary to appreciate that the obliquity of its visual field allows total exploration of the joint and, in particular, of those areas which would otherwise be inaccessible to direct vision.*

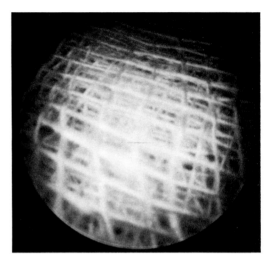

Figure 1.4. *Ordinary gauze observed using the arthroscope. The magnification is proportional to the distance from the end of the arthroscope to the material.*

not allow a very rapid flow. The sheath is provided with two trocar introducers, one sharp and one blunt, for initial entry into the joint.

It is important that the sheath should be slightly longer than the delicate telescope in order to protect its tip. This is essential if the life of the instrument is to be ensured, for minor trauma to the end is inevitable, especially in operative work and even more so if motorized apparatus is used (Fig. 1.5).

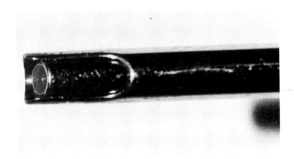

Figure 1.5. *The arthroscope sheath should be longer than the telescope in order to ensure its protection.*

2. Illumination system

This comprises a light source and a connecting cable to the arthroscope. Different types of light sources include xenon, tungsten and arc etc., (Fig. 1.6); the intensity must be adapted to the specific technique used. Thus, for arthroscopy by direct vision, 150 W suffice; while for video arthroscopy, 250 W is usually required according to the sensitivity of the camera used. For photography, the aperture must correspond to that of the arthroscope and the shutter speed must therefore vary according to the light intensity. The shutter exposure should be sufficiently rapid to avoid blurring as a result of movement and requires at least a 250 W light source. Some light sources are augmented by a flash system.

Whatever the maximum light source, it is necessary to be able to vary this during the examination. The intensity required varies according to the structure being examined; thus, for articular cartilage, the reflecting nature of the surface necessitates less light, whereas inside the suprapatellar pouch a higher light intensity is needed.

The colour temperature varies according to the type of light source and is expressed in degrees Kelvin. A tungsten source corresponds to 3200 K, whereas full daylight amounts to

source. During manipulation of the cable it is necessary to avoid folding it too sharply, since this would risk the life of the delicate fibres inside.

It is easy to examine the condition of the cable. If the end normally attached to the light source is illuminated by a lamp, the other extremity may exhibit patchy dark areas, indicating that some of the fibres have ruptured. The extent of such shadowed areas indicates how many of the cable fibres have become fatigued.

3. Video system

A video camera connects to a monitor screen and perhaps to a video recorder.

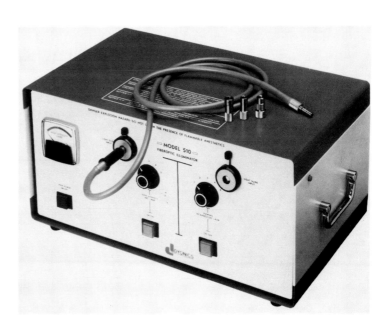

Figure 1.6. *Dyonic light source with a flexible cable and two apertures: one for direct vision arthroscopy and the other for video arthroscopy and photography.*

5400 K. It is necessary to take colour temperature into account in the choice of photographic film so as to achieve proper colour-rendering, otherwise photographs will be too blue or too red.

A flexible cable containing glass or liquid fibres conducts the light from its source to the arthroscope. The overall diameter of the cable must correspond to the intensity of the light

Video colour cameras have been miniaturized so as to weigh less than 200 g (Fig. 1.7). Two types of camera are available. One incorporates a receiving television tube and sensitivity can amount to 10 lx with a greatly enhanced quality of images produced; there is, however, the disadvantage of sensitivity to mechanical shock, and such cameras must be treated with great care. The other type of camera has no

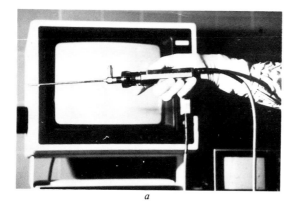

a

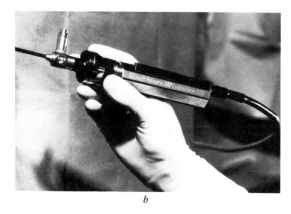

b

Figure 1.7. *Storz camera with television tube. Weight 160g, sensitivity 10lx.*

such fragile tube and is of smaller size. It is more robust, but its sensitivity is less than that of the former type.

The advantages of the more sensitive cameras are that they permit a better exploration of poorly illuminated zones and that they require less light intensity, thereby prolonging the life of both the flexible cable and the arthroscope itself; deterioration in the transmission quality of the cable is inevitable, but is slower with the more sensitive camera.

Cameras incorporate a control, sometimes automatic, in order to adapt to the colour temperature of the light source.

For the display, a 36 cm television screen is a suitable size and should incorporate light intensity, contrast and colour controls.

A video recorder is an advantage, although not indispensable; the three-quarter inch

UMATIC is preferable. This professional format in contrast to the one-half inch size has two advantages: the quality of the images is generally better, especially for large audiences, and it offers better editing facilities.

4. Non-motorized instruments

The following is a list of instruments which we currently use:

> Arthroscopy hook (Fig. 1.8)
> Basket forceps—straight—2.5 and 4.5 mm diam.
> Basket forceps—angulated 90°
> Basket forceps with suction commencement—straight, Dyovac (Fig. 1.9)
> Arthroscopy scissors—straight and 60° angled
> Grasping forceps (Fig. 1.10)
> —meniscal
> —discal (diam. 6 mm)
> Arthroscopy knife with disposable blades (straight, curved, and retrograde) (Fig. 1.11)

This list has been chosen according to a number of criteria: The basket forceps (Fig. 1.12) is the most frequently used instrument; in most cases it has replaced the use of straight scissors since it allows removal of the fragment at the same time as cutting. Both the direction in which it cuts and the depth of cut are controlled.

An arthroscopy knife must be used with great care; there is a temptation to use the tibial plateau as a cutting block when a meniscus is being severed, which risks damaging the articular surface. We use the knife with great restraint. It must be sharp and therefore disposable blades are preferable.

The discal meniscectomy forceps are best for traction because their hold is better than the meniscal type of forceps. Similarly, they can be used for removing osteocartilagenous material in preference to basket forceps, which are more fragile.

The overall shape of the instrument is important: once it has been introduced into the knee, it may not be possible to alter its direction; the shape of the instrument must be suited to the confines of the space allowed. A straight instrument is the basic type, but curved

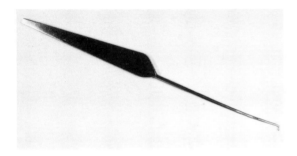

Figure 1.8. *An arthroscopy hook is an indispensable instrument. For diagnosis, it allows study of the lesion not only by vision but also by systematic palpation. For treatment, it allows judgement of the extent of a lesion, the stability of a meniscal wall, etc.*

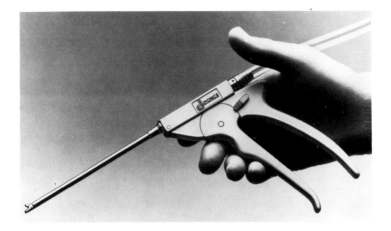

Figure 1.9. *Dyonic resection instrument incorporating aspiration. Constant aspiration allows progressive evacuation of fragments liberated from the structure being operated upon.*

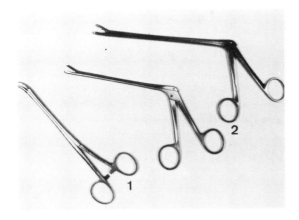

Figure 1.10. *Grasping forceps: 1. Wolf meniscus forceps 2. Disc forceps—these have the advantage of solidity and strength for traction.*

patterns (Fig. 1.13) have advantages such as access around the convexity of the femoral condyle in order to reach a posterior meniscal segment. In fact, the latter are seldom required if care is taken to choose an appropriate port of entry, and this can be assessed as a preliminary measure by probing with a needle so as to evaluate the disposition of the femoral condyle.

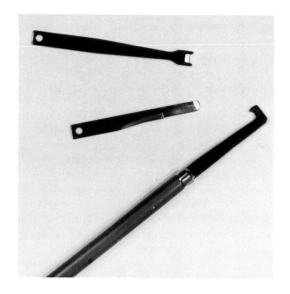

Figure 1.11. *Arthroscopy knife with assorted disposable blades. The handle is straight and cylindrical, allowing introduction into the joint through a 4.5 mm diam. cannula.*

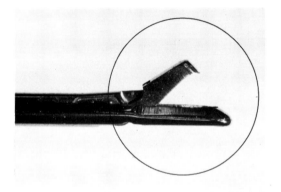

Figure 1.12. *Basket forceps.*

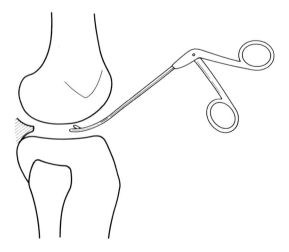

Figure 1.13. *Curved forceps are rarely necessary if the instrument is introduced sufficiently low in order to allow direct access to the posterior segment of the meniscus.*

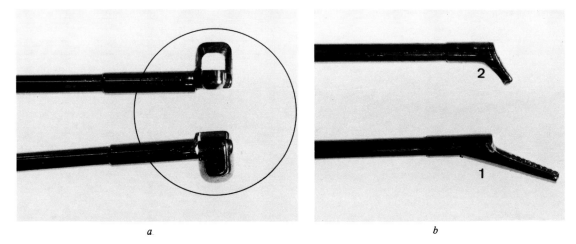

Figure 1.14. *Acufex angulated instruments. (a) 90° angulated blade; (b) 20° (1) and 60° (2) angulated scissors.*

Instruments angulated at the end (Fig. 1.14) are more desirable, for they allow an adequate lateral application despite a tangential approach by the shaft of the instrument.

Strength and solidity are also important criteria, as any operator who has had to search for a broken fragment of an instrument will know! Thus, noting the differences in design of instruments, two points should be observed assiduously: it is obvious that small instruments are likely to be the more fragile, therefore never use a small one where a larger one can be inserted; also, never exert excess force on an instrument which does not cut readily, in case it should fracture.

5. Motorized apparatus

Motorized apparatus includes the shaver as well

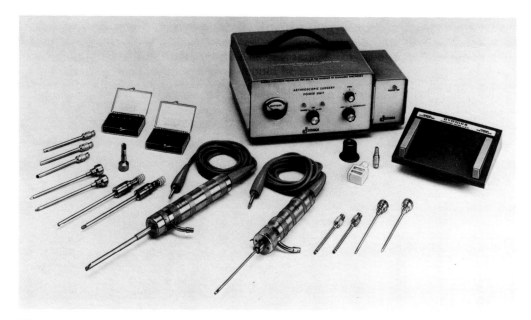

Figure 1.15a. *'Shaver' and 'arthroplasty system'.*

as other arthroplasty systems (Fig. 1.15a). For the shaver, we use three types of blade (Fig. 1.15b):

The synovial resector   is particularly effective against synovial membrane and pathological articular cartilage, especially when it is fibrillated. We prefer the 5.5 mm models.

The cutter   uses the same principles as the shaver by sectioning tissue fragments which can be removed by suction through the blade. It differs, however, in its angle of attack, which is about 45° as opposed to the tangential cut of the shaver, and in its greater efficiency on certain structures, the menisci in particular. Like the shaver, the cutter is proportionally more efficient according to the irregularity or fragmentation of the tissue to be removed. A diameter of 5.5 mm is again our preference.

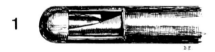

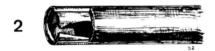

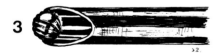

Figure 1.15b. *The three cutting ends usually used are: synovial resector (1) cutter (2) and burr (3).*

The reamer   is enclosed in a sheath which allows both protection and aspiration of fragments removed. The form of the teeth renders the cutting action more aggressive in one direction than in the other.

Two electric motors supplied by a rechargeable battery can rotate the cutters in opposite directions. Effective use demands adequate

irrigation and an accurately controlled suction system. If suction is insufficient, a shaver becomes ineffective, whereas if it is too vigorous, visual access may be lost due to collapse of the inside of the joint with the formation of blebs or bleeding. Regular maintenance is essential, with cleaning and lubrication carried out according to the instructions of the manufacturer.

6. Accessories

The irrigation system   is connected to two sachets of saline, each containing two or three litres. A large caliber tube with a Y-connection, such as is used in urology, terminates in a 4.5 mm diam. cannula inserted into the suprapatellar pouch (Fig. 1.16). Adequate flow is essential and depends on a large bore system.

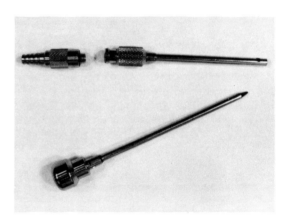

Figure 1.16. *Cannula for admission of irrigating fluid, including mandrel and connection. A diameter of 4.5 mm allows adequate irrigation.*

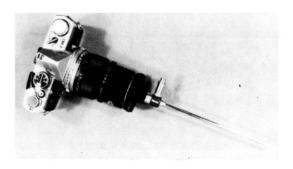

Figure 1.17. *Camera with 135 mm lens coupled to the arthroscope.*

A stirrup or saddle   placed around the tourniquet supports the thigh firmly. It must be robust and simple to manage.

For photography   (Fig. 1.17), automatic shutter exposure and through-lens viewfinding are necessary; a 135 mm focal length lens permits as large an image as possible without exceeding the limits of a 35 mm film. An adapter for the attachment of the arthroscope is necessary. Usually, colour film is used and the film speed should be sufficient to allow a fast shutter speed so as to avoid blurring from movement. The whole field of the 35 mm format is not used and the image appears as a circle inside the rectangle. When setting the camera's film speed, this should be taken into account: for example, if a 400 ASA film is used, the control dial should be set at 800 ASA. The choice between daylight and artificial light film depends on the colour temperature of the light source, but it is possible to adapt an unsuitable film by interposing a filter. It should also be remembered that the light cable itself can alter the colour temperature.

Because of the numerous parameters and variations, it is often necessary to experiment to decide on the appropriate film, the need for a filter, and the adjustment for film speed in order to obtain the best colour rendering.

Instruments must be sterilized according to the manufacturers' recommendations, bearing in mind that a rapid turnover is necessary in order to use the same instruments in one arthroscopy session. For this reason, sterilization by immersion in disinfectant (Cidex, a glutaraldehyde) is currently used.

2

Preparation

Arthroscopy should be performed in the operating theatre, with all the precautions taken for an orthopaedic procedure, despite the apparently minor character of the operation. Careful pre-operative preparation is necessary; the hair around the knee should be removed and the skin checked for blemishes.

1. Anaesthesia

General anaesthesia is advised. It allows a complete examination of the knee in a relaxed state (Fig. 2.1). This should be performed systematically whatever lesion may be suspected. Clinical examination of the opposite knee offers an essential means of comparison.

During the clinical examination under general anaesthesia, it is important to detect losses of flexion and extension, any collateral laxity, the presence of a Lachman sign and the effect thereon of internal or external rotation of the tibia, and the presence of an anterior or posterior drawer sign. Rotatory testing may reveal a click, poorly detected with the patient awake, and this directs attention to the likelihood of a previously unsuspected meniscal lesion, or, sometimes, of a chondral defect.

Regional epidural technique is undoubtedly a useful alternative to general anaesthesia. The choice can be left to the anaesthetist.

Local anaesthesia has been advocated by other arthroscopists.

2. Positioning

The advantages of two important facilities should be considered:

• Exsanguination and a tourniquet, which ensures optimal vision
• An arthroscopy support, which allows full movement of the knee as well as easy valgus and varus stressing of the joint.

(a) ***The opposite limb*** should be positioned in full abduction to allow easy access to all parts of the knee being investigated. In the case of bilateral arthroscopy, the two limbs can be prepared, the second tourniquet being inflated at the end of the first procedure.

(b) ***Exsanguination*** can be performed by elevating the limb for a few minutes, or by the use of an Esmarch bandage, before inflating the tourniquet.

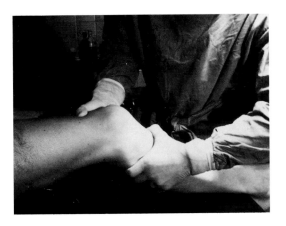

Figure 2.1. *Examination under general anaesthesia. The Lachman test.*

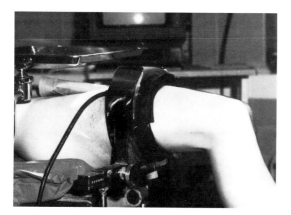

Figure 2.2. *Tourniquet enclosed in the arthroscopy stirrup.*

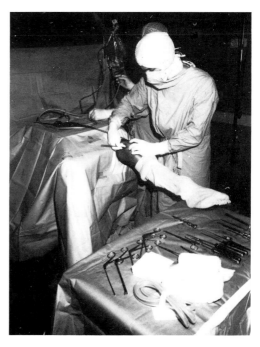

Figure 2.3. *Stockinette applied. The foot rests on the instrument table. Arthroscopy begins by puncture of the suprapatellar pouch.*

(c)   The tourniquet is positioned at the same level as the arthroscopy support, usually at a level 7–10 cm above the upper border of the patella with the knee extended (Fig. 2.2). The length of time during which the tourniquet remains inflated should not exceed one and a half hours.

In order to explore the patella through a superior port of entry, the tourniquet needs to be placed a little higher than usual. If an extra-articular ligamentoplasty using fascialata is performed, the positioning of the tourniquet should be very high. The tourniquet should be inflated *before* positioning it in the arthroscopy support; failure to do this results in pressure being exerted against both the thigh and the support so that later, during the operation, a fall in pressure may be observed.

(d)   The arthroscopy support should surround the tourniquet. Its main advantage is in resisting valgus and varus stressing, thus facilitating the opening of whichever compartment is being explored. The security of the fixation of the stirrup cannot be overemphasized. During movements of the knee, it is very easy for displacement to occur; this can be avoided by application of a Velpeau bandage around the whole. It is well worthwhile checking the solidity of mechanical control before commencing operation.

(e)   Skin sterilization is performed with the usual antiseptic fluids.

(f)   Draping. It is preferable to use disposable sheets which offer a double advantage: they are secure and impermeable. A stockinette extending from the foot to the adhesive on the drape soaks up any spilled fluid which may otherwise trickle on to the feet of the operator (Fig. 2.3).

3. Arthroscopic equipment

The optical system

It is essential to clean the arthroscope. Small droplets of fluid on the optical surface of the eyepiece, as well as distorting the vision transmitted to the video camera, can gradually vaporize and cause progressive mistiness and impede ease of procedure; the eyepiece must be absolutely dry. The quality of the optical surface at the end of the arthroscope should also be checked routinely and if it has a fragmented appearance, the life of this instrument is certainly limited.

The camera can be sterilized by various disinfecting fluids according to the advice of the

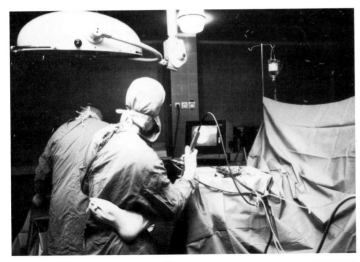

Figure 2.4. *Use of a television system improves comfort for the operator.*

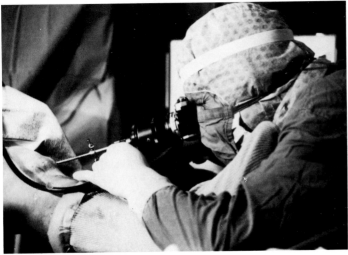

Figure 2.5. *Photography in progress. The operator holds the optical system in one hand and the camera in the other.*

manufacturer, but we prefer to cover the camera in a sterile stockinette drape in order to diminish the inevitable aging of the instrument; all disinfectants are corrosive to some extent. This method also has the advantage of not steaming up the optical surfaces, since it is difficult to achieve complete dryness of the camera after its immersion. The stockinette can be covered by plastic film, which prevents any ingress of fluid during the procedure.

The optical cable

This contains fibres that are very fragile. The path to the operative site must avoid torsion and folding, and the cable should be held in place in such a manner that it will not slide to and fro. The light source should be opposite the

monitor screen; that is to say, on the same side as the limb being investigated.

The monitor screen

This is usually situated on the opposite side of the limb being examined, although some operators prefer it in front of them at the patient's head. The ideal arrangement is to have the screen mounted on a mobile platform so that it can be positioned wherever is most convenient throughout the operation.

The video recorder

This is connected to the television system and the operator can control the recording by

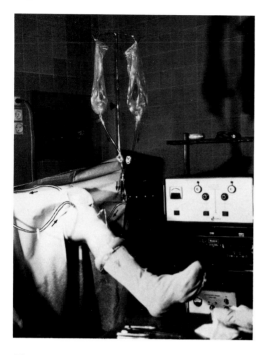

Figure 2.6. *Sachets of physiological saline are suspended at a height which relates to the diameter of the tube. Saline enters the knee through the admission cannula.*

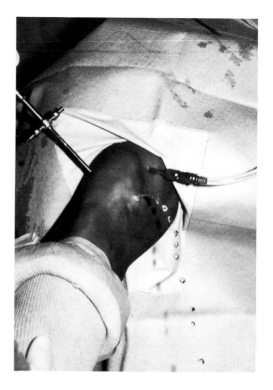

Figure 2.7. *The admission cannula is situated at the superomedial angle of the patella.*

means of a simple pedal switch. The advantages of the video arthroscopy apparatus apply to the operator as well as to the overall operating team. For the operator, the principles of asepsis are much easier to observe. Comfort is ensured, because the operator may remain seated in an optimal position with access to the different compartments of the knee, in particular the posterior regions, and does not have to adopt any uncomfortable posture (Fig. 2.4). Taking video-recorder shots simply involves operating the foot pedal control (Fig. 2.5). It should be noted that photography using a camera is comparatively more complicated and may necessitate a supplementary arthroscope. It is possible for the whole team to follow the operative procedure and foresee what requirements the operator may have. This prevents boredom and creates interest.

The irrigation system

Sachets of physiological saline are connected to the cannula (Fig. 2.6). The flow to the cannula

is determined by two parameters:

—*the pressure*, which is adjustable according to the height of the reservoir; the operator can determine this according to need;
—*the size of the connecting tube* which must not be in any way kinked or constricted.

We prefer to insert the cannula into the superomedial aspect of the suprapatellar pouch at the level of the upper border of the patella (Fig. 2.7). Other arthroscopists prefer the irrigation to enter along the sleeve of the arthroscope, but we think that this technique does not provide a sufficient flow.

The outflow of irrigating fluid can be maintained either through the arthroscope itself or by means of another cannula of sufficient diameter (Fig. 2.8). It is of no advantage to exert suction on this outflow cannula, because sometimes this induces bleeding in the joint. The outlet cannula drains into a bucket or receiver and the arrangement of the drapes prevents flooding.

The aims and advantages of the irrigation system described depend upon a free flow of

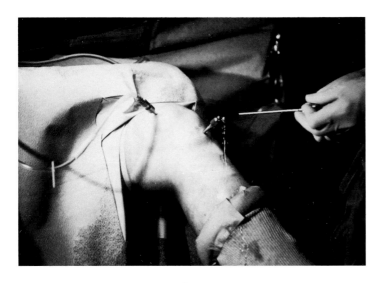

Figure 2.8. *A cannula placed and used as an entry orifice for instruments. This allows evacuation of lavage fluid.*

fluid without the need for high pressure. However, some degree of intra-articular pressure is an advantage, in that this allows access to certain compartments: notably the suprapatellar pouch and the posterior regions; at the same time, it tends to push the folds of synovial membrane out of the way of the arthroscope, thereby improving vision, which can sometimes be impaired.

Free flow of fluid permits lavage which eliminates meniscal or cartilagenous debris and clears any blood or iodized fluid. Lavage also seems to have some therapeutic effect in its own right, and in some cases of arthrosis there has been an improvement in clinical symptoms after arthroscopy, with no other operative intervention. Lavage also reduces the risks of infection.

Problems with irrigation

i. Failure to distend the knee after insertion of the cannula. This may be due to it not being in the suprapatellar pouch, or to the existence of a complete superior plica; the latter is very exceptional and in that case it is necessary to use the arthroscope as the inlet source for initial irrigation distension, after which a second cannula is inserted under direct

vision; this can then be used as the outflow cannula.

ii Insufficient distension and irrigation of the knee. The causes may be several: the sachet may be empty or the tube may become kinked; the height of the sachet may be insufficient, the entry cannula may be partly obscured by a synovial fold, or, the communication within the suprapatellar pouch may be obstructed by tension in the knee joint, a consequence of a particular positioning.

Several solutions may be tried: the inlet pressure may be increased by elevating the sachet or by manual pressure; sometimes a blood transfusion compression bag can be used to advantage. It may be useful to stress the knee into valgus or varus thereby allowing the fluid to pass from the suprapatellar pouch into the tibiofemoral compartments. Finally, it may be useful to reverse the flow, using the arthroscope as the entry and the suprapatellar cannula as the outflow.

iii Deficient outflow. This may be due simply to the sleeve of the arthroscope becoming blocked by meniscal or synovial debris and can be solved by withdrawing the scope and cleaning the sleeve; alternatively, the port of entry chosen may offer an indirect course along a synovial margin which tends to block the sheath at its end; a more direct site should be chosen.

In conclusion, it should be emphasized that careful preparation and setting up of the instrumentation, the video system, and the irrigation technique are all essential prerequisites to successful arthroscopy.

3

Ports of entry

The correct site of entry into the knee is an essential which determines the smooth progress of the entire arthroscopic operation (Fig. 3.1); correct positioning ensures complete vision. Arthroscopic surgery is possible only if the instruments can be introduced easily; it is necessary to consider the angle of attack in order to be precise.

It is convenient to group ports of entry into those that are used most commonly (*primary ports of entry*), those that are used for special types of access (*secondary ports of entry*), and those that may be selected by the operator during the procedure in addition to the main port of entry chosen at the start of the procedure (*complementary ports of entry*).

Primary ports of entry

These comprise the inferior anteromedial and anterolateral approaches. Their positioning is easy and relates to the position of the patellar tendon, the femoral condyles and the tibial plateaux.

1. Anterolateral port

This is identified with the knee flexed between 30° and 60° and by palpating the patellar tendon, the lateral femoral condyle, and the lateral tibial plateau. Having identified these, an incision is made in the angle between the femoral condyle and the patellar tendon; some operators choose to make a vertical and others a horizontal incision. The skin and the subcutaneous tissues are incised. Using the sharp

trocar in the arthroscope sheath, the tissues are penetrated as far as the synovial membrane and then, using the blunt trocar, the joint is entered either by the suprapatellar pouch, the knee being extended, or by the medial compartment. The trocar is then replaced by the telescope.

Using this approach, it is possible to explore the suprapatellar pouch, both medial and lateral compartments, the intercondylar area and, after

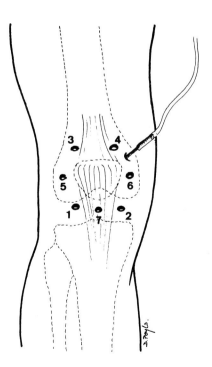

Figure 3.1. *The ports of entry: 1. anterolateral; 2. anteromedial; 3. superolateral; 4. superomedial; 5. lateral parapatellar; 6. medial parapatellar and 7. transpatellar tendon.*

crossing this space, the posteromedial aspect of the knee. When a lateral meniscus lesion is suspected, the point of anterolateral entry can be modified: it should be made a little lower and laterally; the lower position allowing better access to the posterior segment while the more lateral position avoids the patellar tendon which can otherwise be damaged. If it is necessary to perform surgery through the anterolateral approach, the arthroscope may be inserted through the anteromedial port. Stressing the knee into varus opens the lateral compartment to the maximum and entails a shift of the cutaneous incision and of the point of synovial puncture, thereby allowing a direct approach to the site of interest.

The introduction of a needle can sometimes be a useful guide as to the optimal site of puncture of the synovial membrane.

2. Anteromedial port

This approach is best for access to the medial compartment and, in particular, allows access to the posterior part of the medial meniscus. It must be located flush with the surface of the

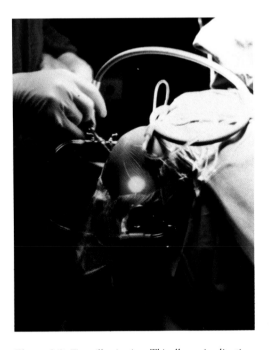

Figure 3.2. *Transillumination. This allows visualization of the neurovascular structures under the skin. (Photograph F. Combelles)*

medial meniscus and parallel to the tibial plateaus near to the patellar tendon, just above the anterior horn. The exact site of puncture can be identified by transillumination with the arthroscope inserted through the anterolateral port. Further, by using this technique, the coincident venous plexus can be identified and thereby avoided (Fig. 3.2). Also, a needle can be used to advantage in order to explore accessibility to the different zones of interest (Fig. 3.3).

Once the position of the needle has been observed, the skin incision may be made correctly, the scalpel blade can be inserted safely just above the meniscus controlled by direct vision; a Kocher forceps can then be used to enlarge the approach at both the cutaneous and the synovial ends. Good access allows easy drainage of fluid, enables evacuation of meniscal or osteochondral fragments, and affords an easy manipulation of the various instruments required subsequently.

This approach is useful for inserting instruments into the medial and lateral compartments as well as into the whole medial collateral recess. It is possible to insert the arthroscope through the same incision, thereby obtaining an excellent view of the lateral compartment as well as of the posterior horn of the medial meniscus, which is otherwise difficult to reach. Again, the posterolateral corner of the knee becomes accessible.

These two approaches facilitate the use of instruments in addition to the arthroscope; they may be changed according to need, although such changes entail loss of time and should be limited. In some cases, an additional puncture is required only in order that the work may be controlled from a different angle; in other cases, it may be indispensable

In general, an instrument inserted on the *same* side of the knee as that requiring attention will allow easier access to the back of the joint, while an instrument passed from the *opposite* side permits work at the front of the joint, the arthroscope, of course, being reversed.

Passage of the arthroscope across the intercondylar space (Figs. 3.4 and 3.5) allows visualization of the posteromedial and posterolateral compartments. The posterior recesses can be visualized from the opposite ports of entry; that is to say, the posteromedial compartment is approached from the anterolateral port and the posterolateral compartment from the anteromedial aspect.

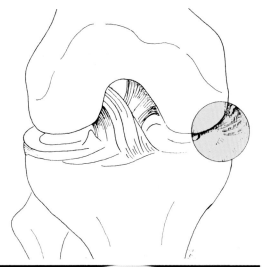

Figure 3.3. *Anteromedial approach. (a) Insertion of needle; (b) puncture with the knife; (c) enlargement by forceps.*

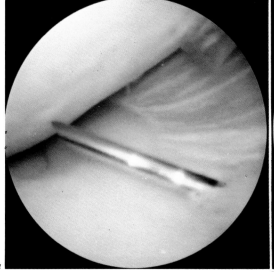

a

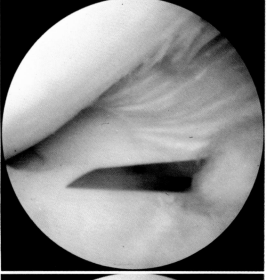

b

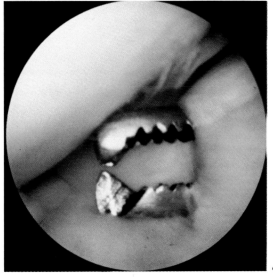

c

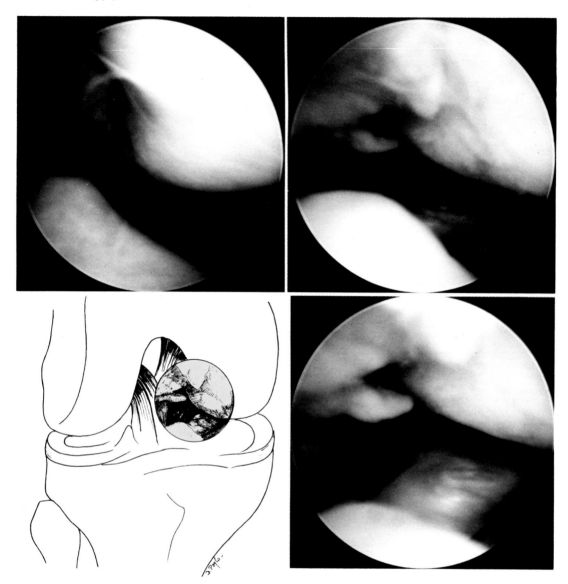

Figure 3.4. *Traverse of the intercondylar area into the posteromedial compartment. The arthroscope is inserted progressively between the plane of the cruciate ligaments and the medial tibiofemoral joint space.*

It may be possible to cross the intercondylar area under direct vision but the passage requires delicacy and may be better performed with the blunt trocar *in situ*; this can then be slid very gently backwards through the interval between the anterior cruciate ligament and the femoro-tibial joint space; a very gentle push will suffice. The knee should be flexed at 90° and great care taken not to perforate the posterior recess on the side being investigated. Sometimes gentle valgus, varus, or rotatory stressing will aid the passage of the instrument. Either side can be approached through the opposite anterior port. The knee should be fully distended and it may be advantageous temporarily to obturate leakage of fluid from around the arthroscope.

Some operators utilize the 70° telescope to great advantage once inside the posterior compartment concerned.

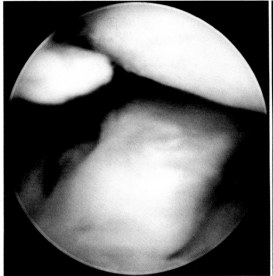 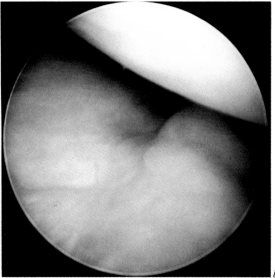

Figure 3.5. *(a) Complated traverse of the intercondylar area. (b) The posteromedial compartment is now seen.*

and this allows the instrument to pass into the suprapatellar pouch.

This technique has certain advantages:

• A direct approach to the intercondylar area is possible because the point of entry is exactly in the centre of the joint.
• There is symmetrical vision of the patellofemoral articular surfaces.
• The possibility exists of using additional instruments passed through two supplementary ports of entry, thereby utilizing in effect three ports.

Among the disadvantages of the transpatellar tendon approach should be included the fact that the tendon never stays exactly in the required position during movements of the knee, and therefore the position of the arthroscope tends to be disturbed; also, it is not usually appropriate to pass instruments for arthroscopic surgery through the tendon.

2. Superior ports of entry

Medial patellar port of entry

The description must be attributed to Patel. The knee is placed in full extension or in very

Secondary ports of entry

1. Transpatellar tendon approach

This has been described by Gillquist. The knee is placed in semiflexion and a point of entry chosen, situated 1 cm below the inferior pole of the patella in the centre of the tendon. The sharp trocar is introduced and then the blunt component follows a lightly ascending trajectory. When the blunt trocar hits the trochlear surface of the femur, extension is completed light flexion and an incision made either medially or laterally in the parapatellar region at the level of the middle of the collateral edge of the patella. These entries allow excellent access to the anterior part of the knee and in particular to the anterior segments of both menisci. Patel himself recognized that there are several blind zones and that the posterior segments of both menisci, in particular the lateral, may be seen only with difficulty. Entry into the intercondylar area is impossible by these routes.

Suprapatellar ports

The knee is placed in complete extension and the suprapatellar area inflated or distended. The entries are situated at the superomedial or superolateral angles of the upper border of the patella. Penetration is easy so long as the knee is well distended and direct vision is possible. These approaches facilitate study of the patellofemoral compartment and allow a perfect assessment of the mating of the patellofemoral articular surfaces. The posterior aspect of the patella can be palpated and the two ports of entry can be used equally well for the passage of instruments. The superolateral port offers direct access to a possible medial plica. Finally, the superior ports of entry can be best for removal of a foreign body, frequently offering a direct approach so that the foreign matter can be grasped and then extracted.

Posterior approaches

Posterior ports are not used routinely, but can prove indispensable in some cases of meniscal pathology (detachment of a posterior segment), ligamentous lesions (especially posterior cruciate), loose bodies, synovial pathology or in the absence of a precise diagnosis.

The first step is to cross the intercondylar area from one of the anterior approaches and then, with the joint flexed from between 60° to 90°, the knee is fully distended with fluid so as to enlarge the posterior compartment. Any leakages of fluid should be sealed temporarily during this manoeuvre. The arthroscope is directed towards the wall of the joint and the operator identifies the angle between the tibial plateau and the condyle and exerts a push which can be identified on the outer aspect of the joint.

A needle is then introduced and passed inwards parallel with the plateau surface a little above it. Its penetration can be checked visually through the arthroscope. Once correctly sited, the usual incision is made with the knife, again under direct vision, and after this has penetrated the joint, the use of Kocher forceps allows entry of a sheath with a soft trocar. After replacing the trocar with the telescope, an arthroscopy hook from the anterior port can be inserted for manipulation and further diagnostic activity.

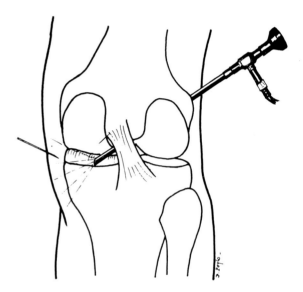

Figure 3.6. *Identification using a needle in order to allow correct positioning of the posteromedial incision. Posterior view.*

Complementary ports of entry

These can be chosen at any time during an arthroscopic procedure if the operator finds that an existing port of entry does not offer correct access. It is a decision which should be taken early and without hesitation, since an inconvenient port of entry augments iatrogenic risk, increases the duration of the procedure, and generally impedes all aspects of the procedure. Sometimes, three ports of entry prove necessary, eg a first for visual access, a second for grasping and a third for cutting.

Problems and ports of entry

(a) Identification can sometimes be difficult in bulky or adipose knees, especially in those with a low patella. This is particularly the case for the anterolateral port.

In cases following previous patellectomy, the condyle and the edge of the tibial plateau are the main identifying landmarks.

Penetration of the joint may be difficult or even impossible, and the possibility of a localized synovial swelling should be considered.

(b) Iatrogenic lesions are possible. A lesion of the articular cartilage can be avoided if one takes the precaution of distending the knee during the anterolateral penetration and visually checking the site of puncture of the anteromedial aspect.

(c) Damage to the anterior horn of the medial meniscus is possible during incision from the anteromedial aspect if this is placed too low. A needle may be used to check the position, thus reducing the risk of error.

(d) A lesion of the venous plexus on the medial side can be avoided by using the transilluminating technique mentioned earlier.

In summary, the two primary ports of entry, if well performed, usually suffice for all problems in the anterior compartments of the knee. Full vision of the posterior compartments necessitates posteromedial or posterolateral ports of entry. Finally, it is necessary to decide *at an early stage* if supplementary ports of entry are going to be required to avoid struggling for access which is obviously difficult.

4

Normal arthroscopic anatomy

The inexperienced observer of an arthroscopy monitor screen is often disorientated by the appearance of the structures. Several factors contribute to the difficulty.

● Distension of the joint by the lavage fluid modifies certain relationships, for example, the enlargement of the suprapatellar pouch and the artificial separation of the patella from its normal trochlear relationship.

● The synovial membrane is looser in certain areas and gives the impression of floating inside the joint.

● Haemarthrosis or joint effusion can blur the image if the lavage flow is insufficient.

● A coupling of the refractive effect of the lavage fluid with the optical system creates a magnification which is exaggerated as the tip of the arthroscope approaches the structure. The magnification is of the order of ×10 at 1 mm and ×2 at 1 cm from the structure observed (Watanabe).

● A 30° oblique telescope introduces a distortion of view which only practice can compensate. This effect is of course significantly greater when the 70° oblique telescope is used.

Arthroscopic technique is very special in that it allows an almost complete exploration of the joint through one approach. It is possible, therefore, to pass from one compartment to another. However, some knees are very 'tight' in that valgus and varus stressing do not allow sufficient widening of the tibiofemoral joint spaces: this can make a complete examination more difficult.

In order to ensure a complete examination of the joint, absolutely clear vision should be obtained and palpation of the intra-joint structures using an arthroscopy hook should be routine. It is absolutely necessary to make a disciplined survey of the joint so as not to miss any pathological entity.

The femoropatellar compartment

The arthroscope can be inserted either through the usual anterolateral port and a hook introduced through an anterior medial incision, or the arthroscope can be introduced through a superior lateral or medial port while the hook is inserted through one of the anterior inferior ports.

The knee is positioned in full extension so that either instrument can be passed easily through the space between the patella and the femur.

The reservoir of irrigating fluid should be positioned high in order to allow adequate distension of the suprapatellar pouch. The operating table can be lowered so as to allow the foot to rest on the instrument table while the operator can remain seated.

The operator begins the exploration by checking the position of the cannula admitting lavage fluid (Fig. 4.1). This is situated above the patella and must be mobile. It is necessary to ensure that the distal extremity of the cannula is not impeded by synovial tissue as this will obstruct free flow and consequent adequate lavage.

The depth of the suprapatellar pouch is variable, sometimes reduced, and may demonstrate an exceptional superior plica, complete or incomplete, a true wall which separates the knee into two cavities (Figs. 4.2 and 4.3).

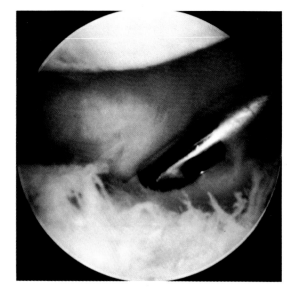

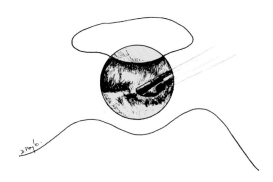

Figure 4.1. *Suprapatellar pouch. The position of the entry cannula for lavage fluid can be identified.*

Sometimes the suprapatellar pouch is very deep and it is necessary to augment the light source intensity in order to visualize it completely, for the synovial membrane absorbs light and darkens all images. The synovial carpet at the margins of the pouch tends to become indistinct, but the junction of the synovial membrane with the trochlear surface of the femur is always clear, presenting the brilliant white appearance of the articular cartilage which contrasts with the pink synovial membrane. Palpation with the arthroscopy hook confirms the visual impression.

More difficult to perceive is the junction between the base of the patella and the synovial membrane along its superior margin. Palpation here is indispensable. It is not always easy when the hook has been inserted through an inferior port.

On the medial surface of the suprapatellar pouch one may find a medial plica. It is frequently minimal in size and it is very rarely

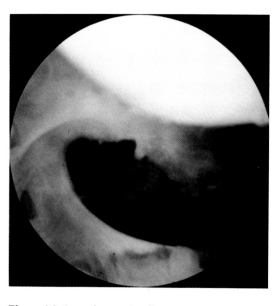

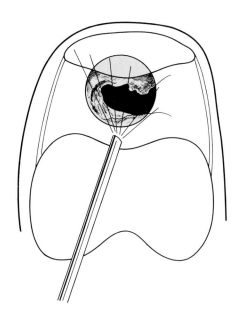

Figure 4.2. *Incomplete superior plica.*

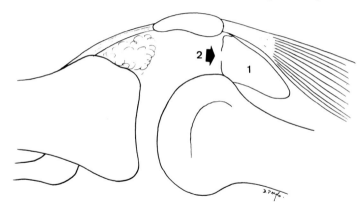

Figure 4.3. *Incomplete superior plica with the knee seen in section.*

pathological (see Chapter 6). It is produced by a simple folding of the synovial membrane which appears horizontal (Fig. 4.4). The beginner must beware of confusing a true plica with a similar appearance that can be produced by air bullae at this level.

The posterior aspect of the patella presents with two sloping surfaces and an intervening crest. This shape is not easy to distinguish clearly in some patients. Paradoxically, it can be difficult to determine exactly where the sloping surface begins or where it meets the crest. The

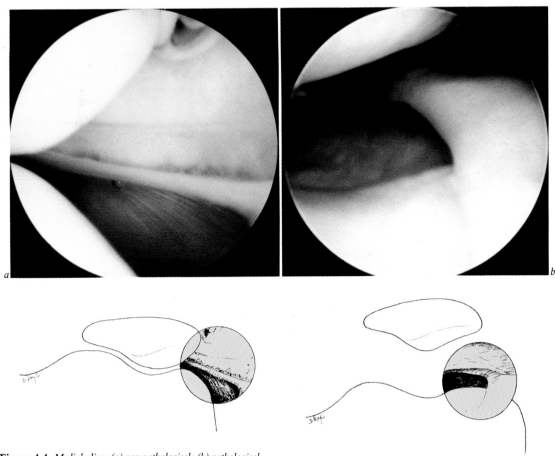

Figure 4.4. *Medial plica: (a) non pathological; (b) pathological.*

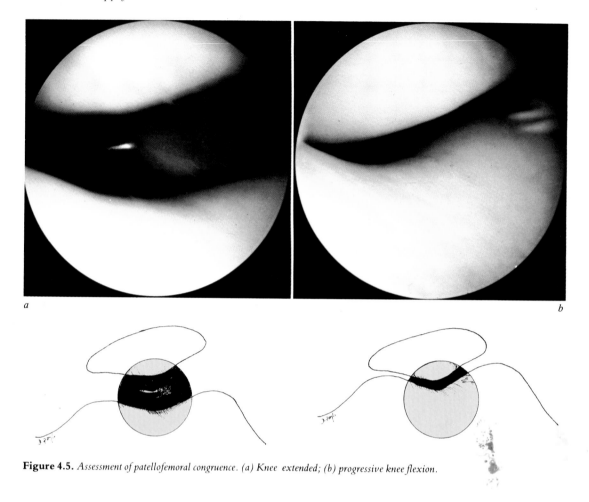

Figure 4.5. *Assessment of patellofemoral congruence. (a) Knee extended; (b) progressive knee flexion.*

line of approach of the arthroscope is important, and associated palpation of the articular surface of the patella is useful.

It is useful to examine the knee during flexion and extension in order to observe whether the crest of the patella coincides with the groove on the trochlear of the femur. The introduction of a needle at the inferior pole of the patella is indispensable in order to verify the position of the cartilage, which can then act as a point of reference. Mobilization of the patella can allow a better view of the two sloping surfaces.

Verification of the inferior pole of the patella is sometimes difficult on account of the proliferation of synovial membrane found there. Introduction of the arthroscope through a superior port is then the best way of ensuring adequate exploration.

The trochlear is usually easy to see and its

groove with the two sloping sides clearly visible.

In order to check the patellofemoral mechanism, it is necessary to flex the knee while gently withdrawing the arthroscope; the trochlear groove can then be visualized as far as the intercondylar area.

If the synovial tissue behind the patellar pouch is too profuse, it may be necessary to use the arthroscopy hook in order to retract it, thereby aiding vision of the trochlear.

The relationship and mating of the patellofemoral surfaces is checked systematically, the arthroscope being placed through an anterolateral port, and its orientation allowing a direct appraisal. If suffices then to flex and extend the knee in order to see if the crest and the groove correspond as they come together (Fig. 4.5). Vision is equally excellent if the arthroscope is introduced through a superior port.

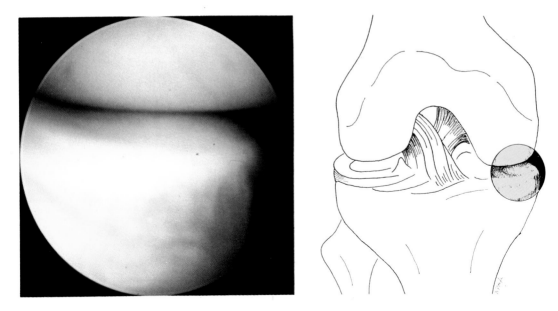

Figure 4.6. *Displacement of the anterior segment of the medial meniscus over the front of the tibial plateau.*

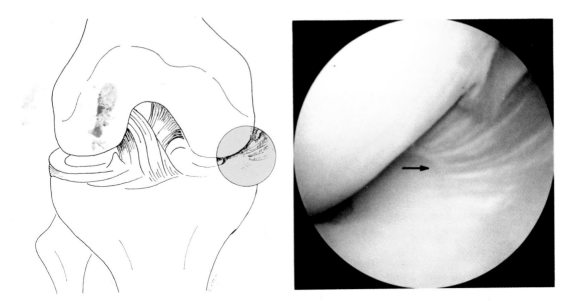

Figure 4.7. *Meniscosynovial junction.*

Medial tibiofemoral compartment

The arthroscope is introduced through an anterolateral port and crosses the knee in front of the intercondylar area in order to visualize the medial compartment. In this position, axial rotation of the 30° telescope allows a complete exploration of the compartment. The knee is lightly flexed in order to relax the medial ligaments, which become tight in full extension. Gentle valgus straining against the arthroscopy stirrup allows slight opening of the medial compartment and facilitates vision. The pressure must be moderate in order to avoid damage to the deep medial collateral ligament, especially in patients of more than fifty years of age.

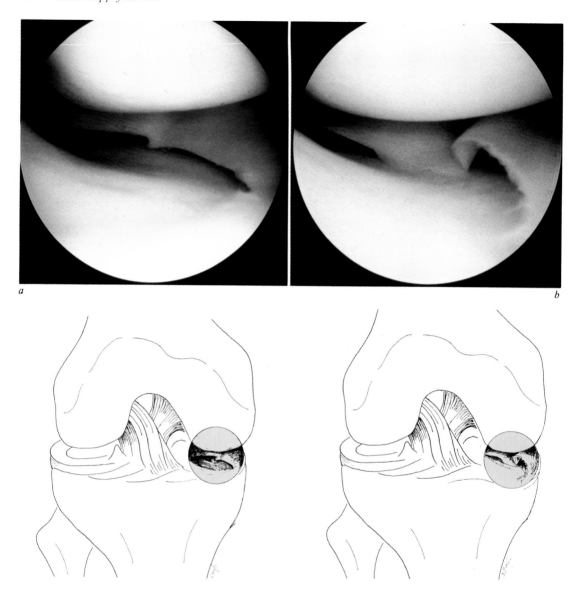

a   *b*

Figure 4.8. *Frilly meniscal margin at the junction of the middle and posterior segment of variable degree.*

The medial meniscus usually presents with an anterior horn which is straight and sometimes slender. It enlarges towards its anterior aspect. Sometimes the anterior segment appears to be sliding off the front of the tibial plateau (Fig. 4.6). It is in the middle segment of the meniscus that the junction with the synovial membrane becomes most clearly delineated (Fig. 4.7). At the junction of the middle and posterior segments, there frequently exists a waviness of the free margin of the meniscus, of varying amplitude (Fig. 4.8). The posterior horn is large and thick and sometimes presents with a small degree of frilliness in front of its attachment. In some cases, visual access is variable; sometimes it is possible to see directly the inferior and superior surfaces of the meniscus as far as the synovial junction, while on other occasions only the superior face is visible and, even then, incompletely.

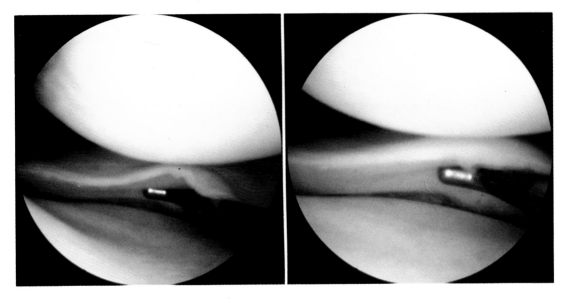

Figure 4.9. *Examination of posterior segment of medial meniscus using an arthroscopy hook. At the same time, the state of the tibial plateau underneath the meniscus can be assessed.*

The zone most difficult to observe is situated at the junction of the posterior horn and the posterior segment.

Palpation with an arthroscopy hook is indispensable as it ensures the absence of any fissures or fractures of the meniscus and helps to check its mobility (Fig. 4.9). Mobility is not great in the case of the medial meniscus, in either its anterior or posterior parts.

The medial femoral condyle is only partially visible with the knee in slight flexion. In order to explore it completely, the knee must be increasingly flexed. This manoeuvre is important because there may be articular cartilage lesions, frequently found in the posterior part.

The tibial plateau is seen directly without particular difficulty with the knee in its lightly flexed position. Palpation with the arthroscopy hook assesses the quality of the articular cartilage.

It is possible to elevate the margin on the meniscus to examine the condition of the articular surface underneath it and, frequently, articular cartilage lesions may be found, especially in the posterior part.

The intercondylar space

The arthroscope is inserted through the anterolateral approach and directed inside, outside or even in front of the anterior cruciate ligament, as appropriate. The knee is flexed to 45° without any valgus or varus stress and the degree of flexion can be varied according to the vision obtained.

The anterior cruciate ligament (Fig. 4.10) presents a variable appearance. Sometimes it is very thick and appears to obstruct the whole notch, while sometimes it is slender, although this has no pathological significance. The direction is oblique passing upwards, backwards and outwards from the tibial attachment. Its superior attachment is often difficult to define exactly. The insertion on the tibia is wide. It is covered by a reflection of synovial membrane on which a fine vascular network is clearly visible. In other cases, the sleeve of synovial tissue is much thicker and it is difficult to define directly the fibres of the ligament itself. It may be possible to distinguish the two fasciculae in this ligament. Palpation of the ligament during flexion and extension, and during performance of the anterior drawer sign

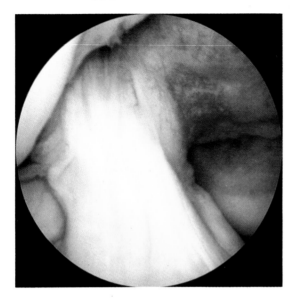

Figure 4.10. *Anterior cruciate ligament.*

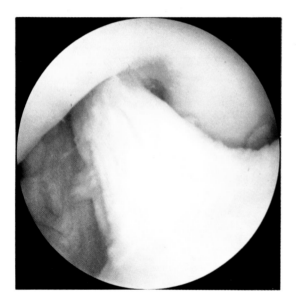

Figure 4.11. *Inferior plica. This can be mistaken for the anterior cruciate ligament.*

is useful in order to define the state of tension if there are any doubts on this point.

Certain circumstances can complicate examination of the anterior cruciate ligament. Often there is an inferior plica (Fig. 4.11); this is also called a synovial infrapatellar plica, ligamentum mucosum, and adipose ligament. It stretches from the floor of the notch to a fatty pad at the inferior pole of the patella. Sometimes its appearance can be confused with that of the anterior cruciate ligament. Moreover, it can be confluent with the anterior cruciate ligament and make assessment of the latter difficult. With the aid of the hook, it is usually possible to separate the inferior plica and find underneath the anterior cruciate ligament itself.

The synovial tissue is frequently hypertrophied in the intercondylar notch and it can be difficult to define the anterior cruciate ligament; palpation is performed blind. If it is absolutely necessary to expose the anterior ligament, it may be necessary to perform a partial resection of the synovial tissue, although this must be performed with great care.

Lateral compartment

The arthroscope is inserted by a medial or lateral port. Change of entry in order to see or palpate a particular segment of the meniscus or articular surface may be necessary. Usually the knee is in light flexion associated with varus stressing; in some cases flexion to as much as 90° may be advantageous.

The lateral meniscus presents a more rounded shape than the medial meniscus (Fig. 4.12). Its anterior horn arises adjacent to the inferior attachment of the anterior cruciate ligament

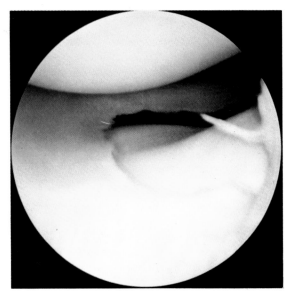

Figure 4.12. *Lateral meniscus. Note the rounded form.*

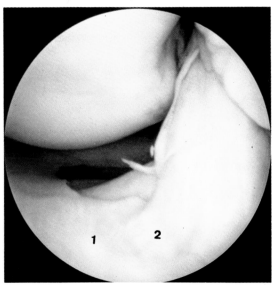

Figure 4.13. *The anterior horn of the lateral meniscus is very close to the tibial attachment of the anterior cruciate ligament. 1. Anterior horn of the lateral meniscus; 2. lower end of the anterior cruciate ligament.*

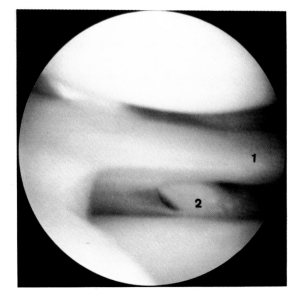

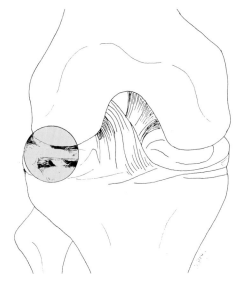

Figure 4.14. *The popliteal hiatus. From this appears the popliteus tendon. 1. Lateral meniscus; 2. popliteus tendon.*

(Fig. 4.13). The anterior segment is wide, thick and of characteristic appearance while the middle segment is also broad and presents a lightly wavy free border. The popliteal tendon hiatus is usually clearly visible and the tendon itself shines brightly in the back of the joint and is easily recognizable (Fig. 4.14). This tendon is orientated downwards and medially. Often, at the junction of the middle segment and of the popliteal hiatus there is a zone of synovial proliferation. The posterior segment and the posterior horn of the lateral meniscus are both wide and thick.

Palpation of the lateral meniscus reveals much greater mobility than is the case for the medial component. This is due to the popliteus

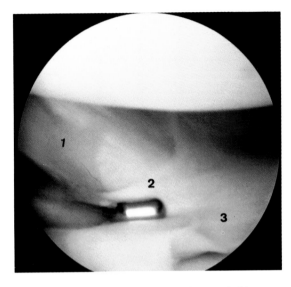

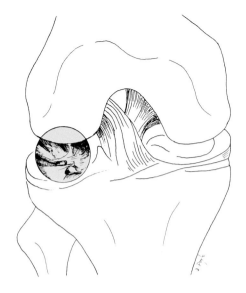

Figure 4.15. *Examination of the popliteal hiatus and of the popliteal tendon using the arthroscopy hook. 1. Popliteal tendon; 2. popliteal hiatus; 3. lateral meniscus.*

hiatus which allows freedom of firm attachment in this area, other than by a meniscosynovial membrane. This mobility, even though considerable, in normal circumstances never allows dislocation of the posterior part of the meniscus; if dislocation can be effected by palpation, there must be a meniscal lesion. Palpation of the popliteal hiatus is essential in order to rule out a rupture of the meniscosynovial attachment (Fig. 4.15). The tension in the popliteal tendon itself can also be checked.

The lateral condyle of the tibial plateau can be examined in the same way as for the medial side, underneath the free margin of the meniscus.

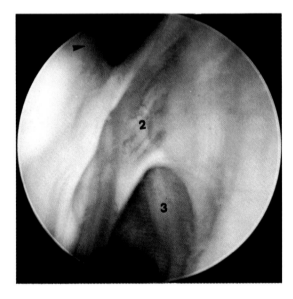

Figure 4.16. *Upper part of the medial collateral recess. 1. (indicated by an arrow) The beginning of the suprapatellar pouch. 2. Synovial reflection. 3. Commencement of the collateral recess.*

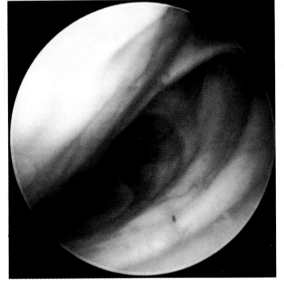

Figure 4.17. *Medial collateral recess.*

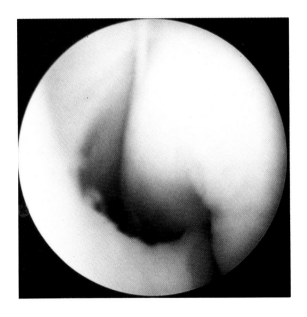
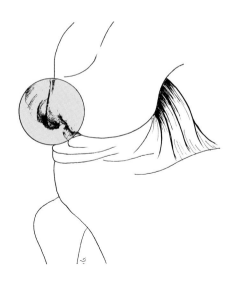

Figure 4.18. *The popliteal tendon seen through the lateral collateral recess.*

The collateral recesses

These spaces can be examined through an ipsilateral port. The knee is in extension or lightly flexed, avoiding valgus or varus stressing which would draw together the walls of the recess and make distension difficult. The synovial layer on the medial and lateral wall of both recesses terminates above and posteriorly in a synovial plica (Figs. 4.16 and 4.17). On the lateral side, passing from the lateral recess, it is possible to observe the popliteal tendon from an angle different from that obtained during exploration of the lateral compartment; that part of the tendon just above its insertion onto the tibia can be seen (Fig. 4.18).

Posteromedial compartment

In order to see the posteromedial compartment, the arthroscope should cross the intercondylar notch on the medial side of the anterior cruciate ligament or be inserted through a posteromedial port. Subsequently, instruments can be passed through whichever port remains free. The knee is flexed to about 90° and it is very important to have maximum distension of the joint by elevating the irrigation system and

reducing outflow. The use of a 70° oblique telescope improves the possibilities of vision. When the arthroscope is passed across the intercondylar notch, the posteromedial cul-de-sac and the medial femoral condyle become visible. The posteromedial approach using the arthroscope clearly identifies the posterior segment and the posterior horn of the meniscus as well as its synovial margin. Also, the posterior cruciate ligament can be seen, but its assessment is always difficult, even with the use of the meniscus hook, because often it is so embedded in synovial tissue.

The posterolateral compartment

As for the posteromedial compartment, the arthroscope can be inserted across the intercondylar notch or directly by a posterolateral port.

The knee is flexed to 90° and, with maximum distension of the joint space, the transcondylar notch approach allows visualization of the posterolateral cul-de-sac and of the lateral condyle of the femur. Only a posterolateral entry, however, allows access to the meniscosynovial junction and a full inspection (Fig. 4.19).

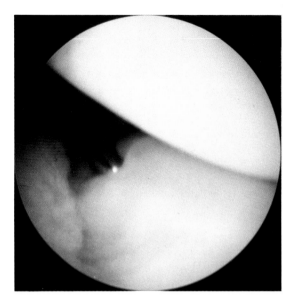
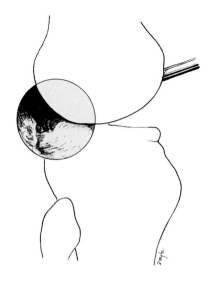

Figure 4.19. *Posterolateral compartment. An arthroscopy hook is seen examining the meniscosynovial junction. The hook has been placed through the intercondylar space while the arthroscope has been introduced through a posterolateral port.*

Conclusion

Only a precise understanding of the normal arthroscopic anatomy of the knee will enable diagnosis of abnormalities, thereby allowing a correct therapeutic procedure.

5

Lesions of the menisci and surgical management

General features

Lesions of the menisci vary according to differing anatomical sites, level and, of course, lateral and medial involvement. An understanding of the different types is essential for the determination of proper therapeutic management and, in particular, as a guide to the necessary extent of resection of a meniscus. They will be classified according to their site in the meniscus and in terms of their anatomical pathology.

For the purposes of arthroscopy, each meniscus can be divided into three equal segments (Fig. 5.1): anterior, middle, and posterior. The anterior and posterior segments are prolonged at their extremities by the anterior and posterior horns, which are insertions of the ends of the menisci onto the tibial plateau.

Three types of rupture can be distinguished (Fig. 5.2).

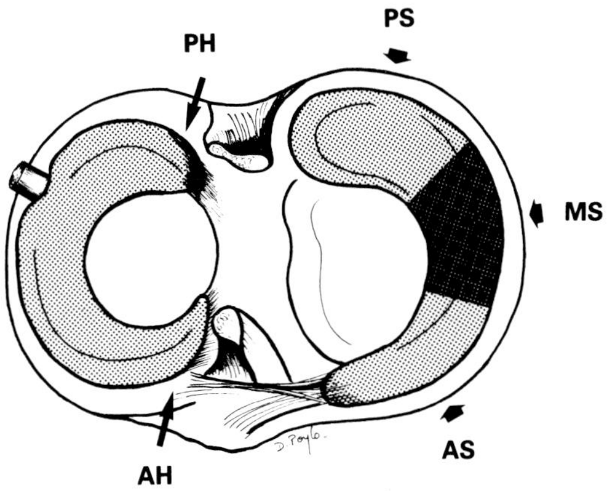

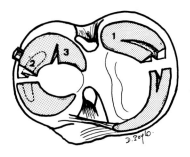

Figure 5.2. *Meniscal lesions. 1. Longitudinal rupture; 2. horizontal rupture; 3. transverse rupture.*

Figure 5.1. *The three meniscal segments. PH = Posterior horn; AH = anterior horn; PS = posterior segment; MS = middle segment; AS = anterior segment.*

i. Longitudinal ruptures are situated in the direction of the longitudinal fibres of the meniscus. The rupture may be vertical in relation to the surface of the meniscus, or oblique. It may be complete, involving the whole thickness of the meniscus or, incomplete, being visible only from the superior or inferior surface (Fig. 5.3). The site may be at a variable distance from the free border of the meniscus, as far peripherally as the meniscosynovial junction.

ii. Horizontal ruptures form a cleavage in the thickness of the meniscus, and it is important to appreciate the depth.

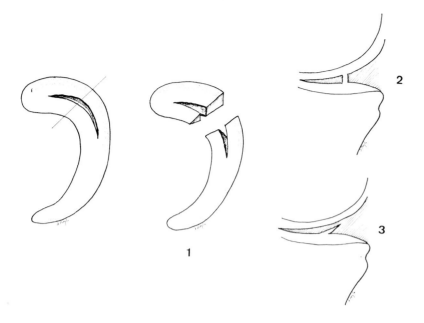

Figure 5.3. *Longitudinal rupture: 1. and 2. complete; 3. incomplete and oblique.*

iii. Transverse ruptures are perpendicular, extending from the free border towards the periphery.

These differing morphological types can present in combination, forming *complex* meniscal lesions.

The overall appraisal of a meniscal lesion must be related to the clinical features that it has caused, and not just to the findings on arthrography and at arthroscopy.

Arthrography

Arthrography constitutes a valuable first measure in diagnosis. Good technique confirms a meniscal lesion in the majority of cases. Moreover, it guides the subsequent arthroscopy towards the lesion. Arthrography is of great importance in demonstrating certain posterior detachments of the menisci, which can be seen only with difficulty at arthroscopy because they are covered by an intact synovial membrane. As previously emphasized, the quality of arthrography must be very high if this method is to be exploited fully.

Arthroscopy

The first aim is to confirm the presence of a meniscal lesion, then to identify its site and its type; visualization alone is not sufficient—it is absolutely necessary to palpate and to explore the lesion using a hook. This will often bring into view some feature which is not visible by simple passive observation, and extended study and assessment of the stability of the meniscus must follow. In certain instances, the operator should not hesitate to use different approaches, which we shall see later are particularly relevant in the posteromedial and posterior lateral compartments.

Operative arthroscopy follows the diagnostic procedure.

The medial meniscus

Of the three types of medial meniscal lesion, the longitudinal type is by far the most frequent. Transverse ruptures are rare. The posterior segment is the commonest site. We have not encountered any anterior lesions other

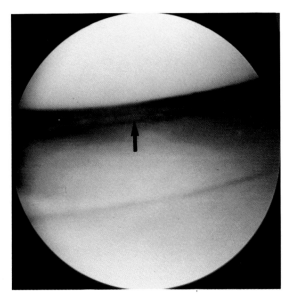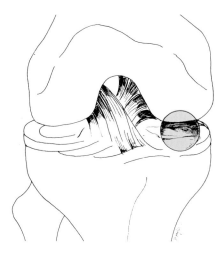

Figure 5.4. *Complete longitudinal rupture of the posterior segment of the medial meniscus.*

than those longitudinal splits which have propagated from the posterior segments.

i. Longitudinal rupture

This may be vertical or oblique and at a variable distance from the meniscosynovial junction (Fig. 5.4). It may pose some problems in diagnosis at arthroscopy for it is not always complete and therefore not visible immediately (Fig. 5.5). Difficulty of identification is commonest when the rupture is incomplete and opens onto the inferior surface and, in such a case, palpation with the arthroscopy hook is particularly important. The hook can, sometimes, first elevate the meniscus and then be introduced gently from beneath, thereby exposing the split, but such direct vision is not always possible. The following manoeuvre may be helpful: the hook is placed on the upper surface of the posterior segment of the meniscus and progressively moved forward while pressing on the surface of the meniscus; when it reaches the site of rupture, it produces a characteristic tilting of the free border as the hook detects the underlying depression.

ii. The tongue or parrot beak lesion

When the longitudinal rupture involves the free border of the meniscus, it can produce one or two tongues (Fig. 5.6) based either at the posterior segment, the posterior horn or in the middle segment. It is less common for the tongue to arise from the whole width of the meniscus. The end of the tongue becomes readily trapped between the tibial and femoral surfaces and therefore tends to become piriform in shape, like the clapper of a bell. Tongues are usually very easy to visualize (Fig. 5.7), but it is important to remember that they can become infolded under the meniscus, or over it in the paracondylar region, and it is always necessary to explore them thoroughly with the arthroscopy hook.

iii. The bucket handle rupture

This comprises an extension of a longitudinal posterior tear, anteriorly (Fig. 5.8). The bucket handle may remain in place so that the arthrographic image is characteristic while, at arthroscopy, the highly mobile nature of the bucket handle can be confirmed by using the hook. The bucket handle may be displaced into the intercondylar area. In this instance, arthrographic diagnosis may be more difficult and the shape of the margin of the meniscus seen may appear merely narrow.

At arthroscopy, the bucket handle is found in the intercondylar notch and can be followed

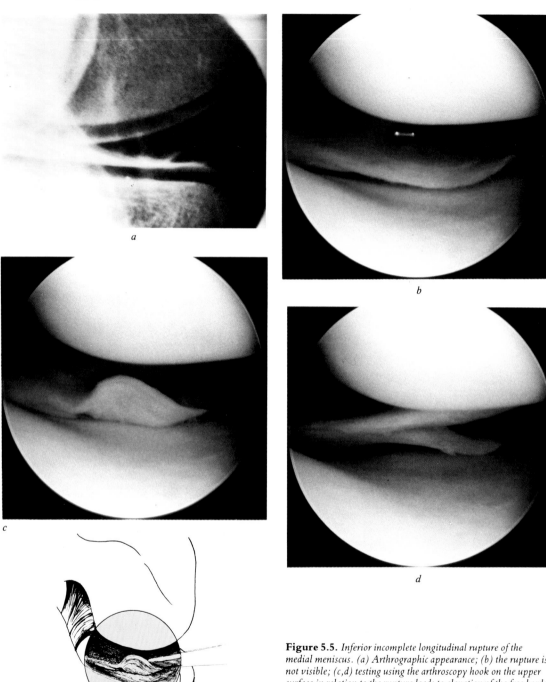

a

b

c

d

Figure 5.5. *Inferior incomplete longitudinal rupture of the medial meniscus. (a) Arthrographic appearance; (b) the rupture is not visible; (c,d) testing using the arthroscopy hook on the upper surface in relation to the rupture leads to elevation of the free border of the meniscus adjacent.*

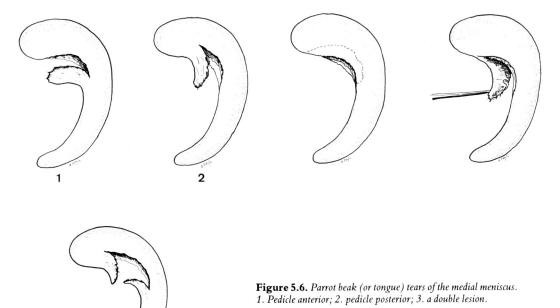

1 2 3

Figure 5.6. *Parrot beak (or tongue) tears of the medial meniscus.*
1. Pedicle anterior; 2. pedicle posterior; 3. a double lesion.

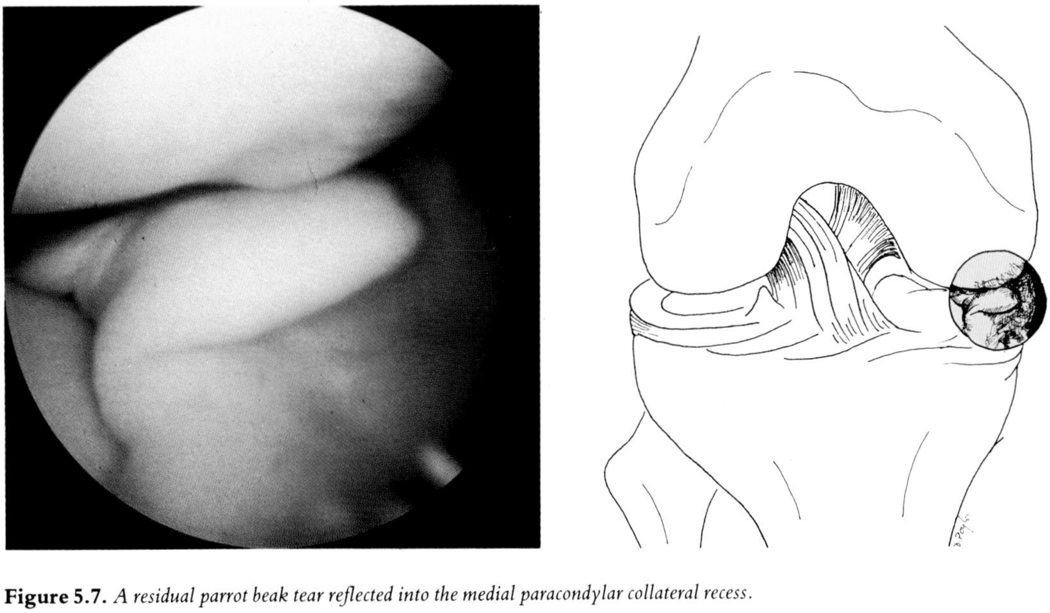

Figure 5.7. *A residual parrot beak tear reflected into the medial paracondylar collateral recess.*

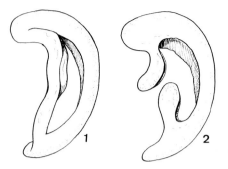

Figure 5.8. *1. Bucket handle tear of the medial meniscus and 2. broken in its middle part.*

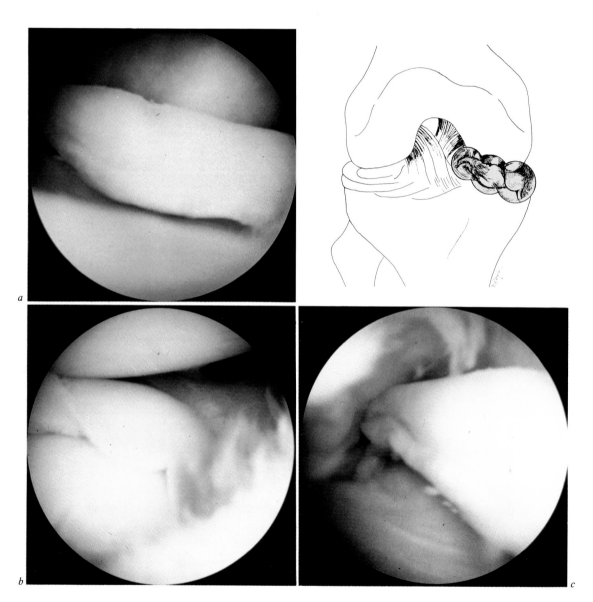

Figure 5.9. *Bucket handle tear subluxed into the intercondylar area. (a) Middle segment; (b) anterior segment at its junction with the remainder of the meniscus; (c) posterior segment, which is impacted in the intercondylar area before rejoining the posterior horn.*

anteriorly towards its junction with the rest of the meniscus. Posteriorly, before reduction of the bucket handle, it seems to lose itself in the intercondylar area (Fig. 5.9). Failure to diagnose the bucket handle tear is an easy trap to fall into. Thus, if the arthroscopist views only the residual margin of the meniscus which is still intact, it can at first sight look like a normal meniscus. Attention should be aroused by its somewhat straight appearance and by the irregularities along the free border or on the inferior surface; it suffices then to withdraw the arthroscope in order to examine the intercondylar area carefully, and the displaced bucket handle will be found.

Two bucket handles can exist, an important point because sometimes only careful probing with the arthroscopy hook after ablation of one bucket handle will avoid missing such a second example.

Finally, the bucket handle can have ruptured spontaneously. This may occur at the posterior attachment leading to a tongue based anteriorly; conversely, the base can be anterior, with the tongue directed posteriorly and often tilted into the posteromedial compartment or maybe into the middle of the joint. Finally, rupture can have occurred in the centre, causing the formation of two long tongues.

iv. Meniscosynovial lesion

The vascular meniscosynovial zone is ruptured in the posterior segment (Fig. 5.10). This occurs more frequently in the medial meniscus

and is associated commonly with a tear of the anterior cruciate ligament. Its diagnosis is particularly important because it is amenable to repair by suture. Arthroscopic diagnosis may be difficult and in order not to miss the lesion, it is necessary to consider its possibility in all examples of anterior cruciate rupture. Palpation with the arthroscopy hook of the posterior segments of the medial meniscus, either through anterolateral or anteromedial ports of entry, is the surest way of discovering a meniscosynovial detachment, since the peripheral site of the detachment can make visualization difficult. While the arthroscopy hook will penetrate into a dehiscence it is sometimes difficult to distinguish this from a normal meniscosynovial recess (Fig. 5.11). The arthroscope can be introduced across the intercondylar notch using, if necessary, a 70° oblique telescope in order to examine fully the

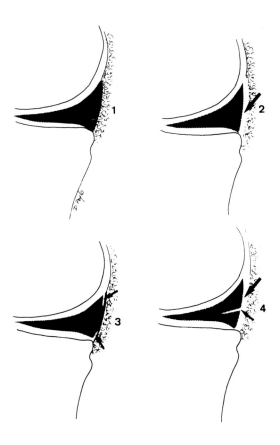

Figure 5.11. *Detachment at meniscosynovial recess. 1. Normal medial meniscus; 2. simple detachment; 3. inferior and superior meniscal recesses; 4. complete detachment with a horizontal meniscal component.*

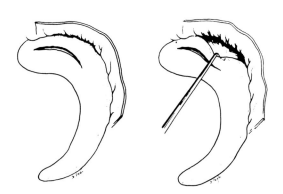

Figure 5.10. *Peripheral detachment of the meniscosynovial junction in contrast with a longitudinal rupture which remains intra-meniscal.*

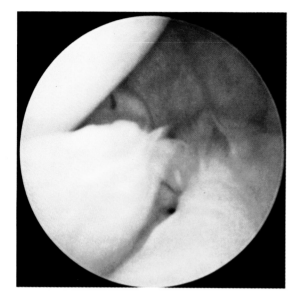
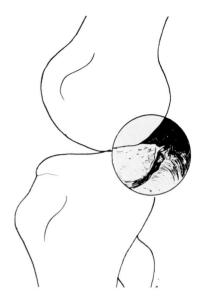

Figure 5.12. *Posterior meniscal detachment as seen through the posteromedial port of entry.*

posteromedial compartment; however, if necessary, the operator should not hesitate to use a posteromedial approach, which will allow direct vision of a possible detachment (Fig. 5.12). Even by the latter approach, the diagnosis may still be difficult if the detachment is incomplete or if it is covered by an intact synovial membrane. Arthroscopy may not demonstrate an association of this peripheral detachment with a horizontal cleavage of the meniscus, a contraindication to repair by

suturing. It is here that arthrography is particularly useful for it may demonstrate very clearly the repairable or non-repairable varieties of lesion (Fig. 5.13).

v. Horizontal rupture

Horizontal ruptures are rare in the medial meniscus. They occur more frequently with cystic degeneration (Fig. 5.14). Cysts may

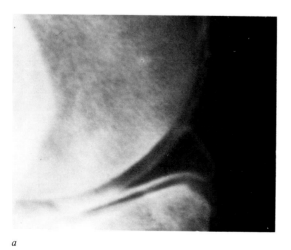

a

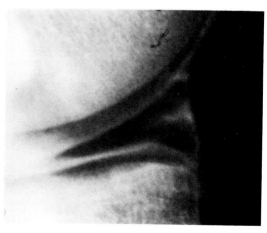

b

Figure 5.13. *Arthrography can be very precise with this type of lesion. (a) Simple detachment; (b) detachment with a horizontal meniscal component.*

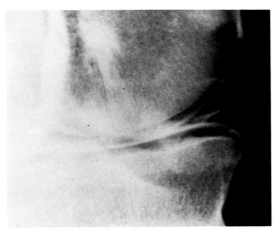

Figure 5.14. *Cyst of the medial meniscus. These are sometimes extensive; here, a horizontal cleavage (easily seen on arthrography) reaching the periphery of the meniscus.*

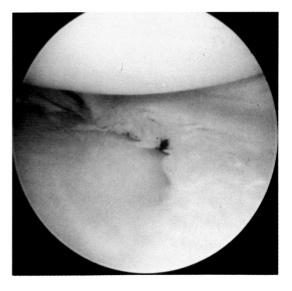

progress in a horizontal direction, reaching the meniscosynovial junction where they may become palpable. Even in the absence of a cyst, a horizontal cleavage in the periphery of the meniscus is sometimes associated with the lesions described earlier and must be sought systematically during a resection to avoid leaving a pathological meniscal remnant.

vi. Transverse rupture

This type of lesion is also rare on the medial side. It is most frequently associated with the onset of degenerative changes, as has been shown by Dorfmann, Boyer and Bonvarlet (Fig. 5.15). At the junction of the middle and posterior segments a rupture occurs, which is transverse or variably oblique. On either side of this lesion, the meniscus presents a degenerative appearance and there are associated articular cartilage lesions on both femoral and tibial surfaces.

vii. Medial discoid meniscus

This is a rare condition presenting an appearance identical to that of the lateral side, and the

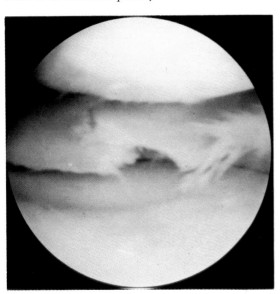

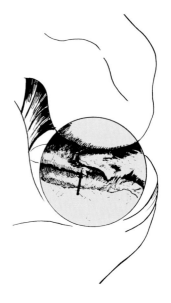

Figure 5.15. *Transverse rupture of the medial meniscus of degenerative origin.*

meniscus covers the entire tibial plateau. It may be complete, incomplete, or it may be ruptured.

viii. Complex lesions

The association of the individual configurations described above can present a complex appearance. This is particularly the case in degenerative meniscosis and a completely systematic description may not be possible. There exists a general softening of meniscal texture associated with numerous fissures, sometimes longitudinal or transverse, together with tongues of varying size. These lesions relate to a generalized osteoarthrosis of the joint. Further development results in progressive lamination of the meniscal structure with separation and the eventual appearance of a straight irregular wall.

ix. Chondrocalcinosis

The meniscus appears to be studded with deposits of calcium pyrophosphate (Fig. 5.16); the consistency is often very hard.

x. Lesions of the meniscal wall after meniscectomy

A meniscectomy, whether performed during arthrotomy or arthroscopically, may not be satisfactory and leave some areas of pathological meniscal wall (Fig. 5.17). Typical examples are a residual posterior tongue or a classic horizontal cleavage—a so-called 'fish mouth'. The most frequent remnant is the superior lip which has been insufficiently resected because of difficult arthroscopic access. Persistence of a projecting angle at the level of the healthy and resected areas of meniscal tissue can be responsible for subsequent deterioration; thus it is always necessary to ensure that such irregularities are smoothed so as to give a harmonious curve, thereby avoiding the formation of a subsequent tongue.

Lateral meniscus

i. Transverse lesions (Fig. 5.18)

These occur more frequently in the lateral meniscus than in the medial side. They extend from the free border more or less towards the meniscosynovial zone and are found most commonly in the middle segment. Usually they consist of a solitary lesion. Sometimes they are the consequence of a meniscal cyst, in which case, palpation with the arthroscopy hook must be systematic and may discover an intrameniscal extension.

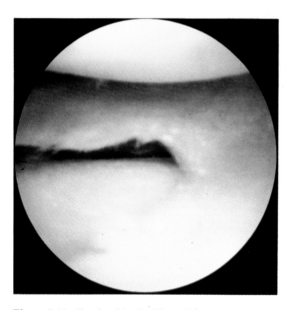

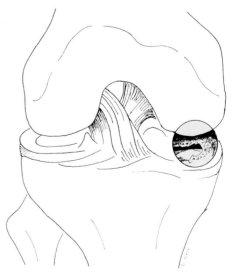

Figure 5.16. *Chondrocalcinosis of the medial meniscus.*

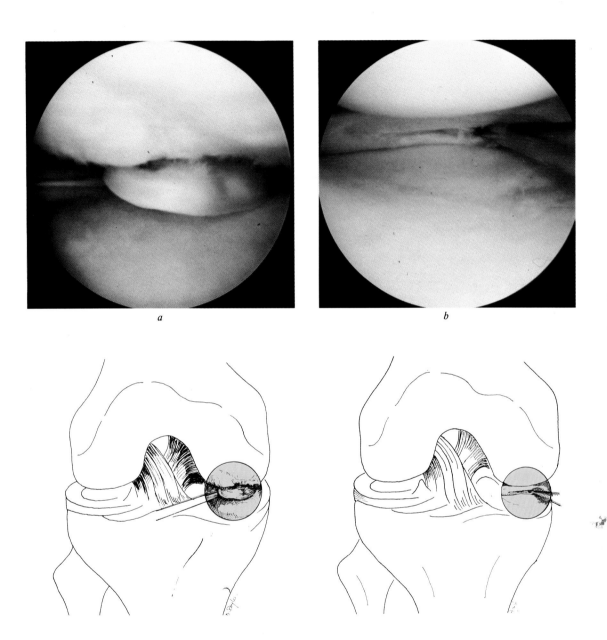

a   *b*

Figure 5.17. *Lesion of the residual meniscal wall after meniscectomy. (a) Persistence of a tongue demonstrated by the hook; (b) horizontal fissure which was left due to an insufficient resection.*

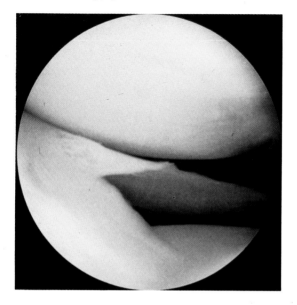

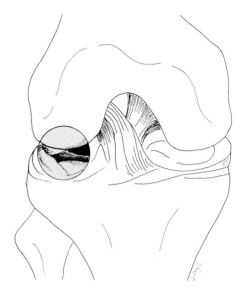

Figure 5.18. *Transverse rupture of the middle segment of the lateral meniscus.*

ii. Longitudinal lesion (Fig. 5.19)

This is the commonest type. It may be posteriorly situated (Fig. 5.20), intrameniscal and at a variable distance from the meniscosynovial junction, often associated with a rupture of the anterior cruciate ligament. Most frequently, it is vertical and may be incomplete, opening onto either the superior or the inferior surface.

Longitudinal ruptures may also be found in the anterior segment, very far forward and sometimes reaching the meniscosynovial junction; arthroscopic diagnosis can be difficult, underlining again the importance of palpation with the hook.

iii. Bucket handle tear (Fig. 5.21)

This is found less frequently on the lateral side than in the medial meniscus. The bucket handle displaces into the condylar area and can sometimes be voluminous. This is especially the case in a ruptured discoid meniscus. Here again, the clinician must be careful not to miss the displaced bucket handle by confusing the residual rim with a 'short' meniscus (Fig. 5.22). Only systematic exploration of the intercondylar area will avoid this mistake.

iv. Tongue (parrot beak)

This is most commonly based in the anterior segment.

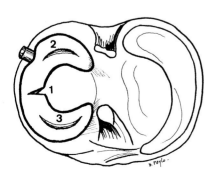

Figure 5.19. *Ruptures of the lateral meniscus: 1. transverse; 2. posterior longitudinal; 3. anterior longitudinal.*

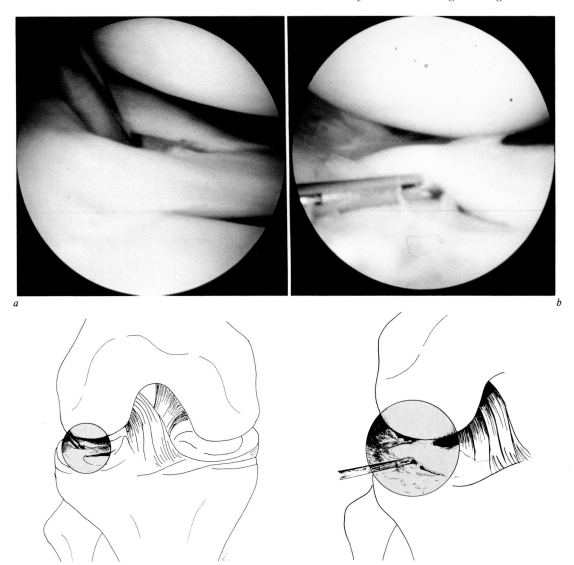

Figure 5.20. *(a) Posterior longitudinal rupture. (b) Anterior longitudinal rupture.*

Figure 5.21. *Bucket handle tear of the lateral meniscus.*

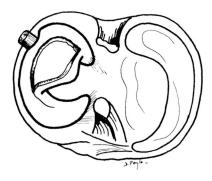

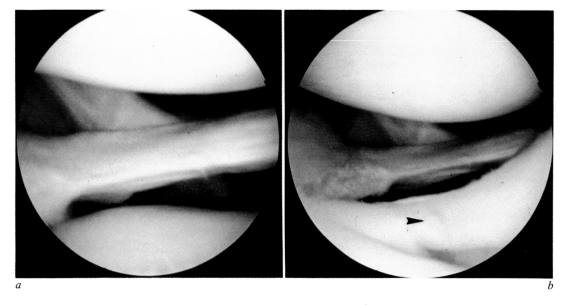

a   b

Figure 5.22. *Bucket handle tear of the lateral meniscus. (a) Residual meniscal wall with the appearance of a normal meniscus; (b) the same meniscus: the bucket handle reflected towards the arthroscope.*

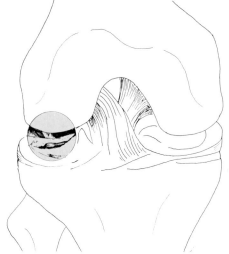

v. Meniscosynovial detachment

Posteriorly, there is a prolongation of the hiatus of the popliteal tendon medially, towards the posterior horn (Fig. 5.23). Arthrographic diagnosis is difficult on account of the superimposition of the images of the popliteal hiatus (Fig. 5.24). Palpation with the hook remains essential in the diagnosis, in searching for the lesion and forward displacement of the mobile posterior segment following traction. When-ever necessary, the arthroscopist should make a posterolateral puncture.

These posterior disinsertions, when partial, explain the condition found in certain 'hyper-mobile' menisci.

vi. Complex lesions

Combinations of different morphological types are difficult to describe and are frequently associated with a degenerative condition.

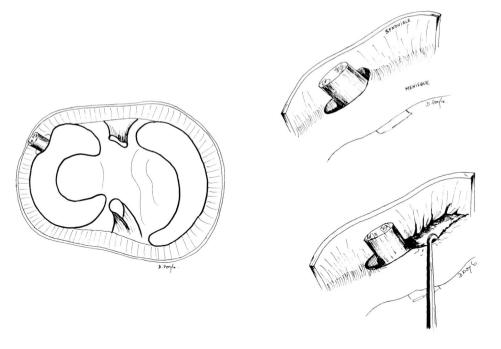

Figure 5.23. *Posterior detachment of the lateral meniscus extending towards the popliteal hiatus.*

vii. Lateral cystic meniscus (Fig. 5.25)

This is a specific condition which associates a meniscal lesion with a cyst, whether the latter is palpable or not. It usually involves the middle segment of the lateral meniscus and, initially, it presents as a simple intrameniscal tunnel (Fig. 5.26) which gradually develops into a horizontal cleavage affecting the meniscosynovial junction anterior to the popliteal hiatus forming a cystic pouch.

Diagnosis is based upon the clinical signs associated with a lateral swelling of variable volume at the level of the tibiofemoral joint space; in typical cases, arthrography demonstrates a horizontal cleavage extending to the periphery, with filling of the cyst; at arthroscopy, all of our cases were associated with a horizontal cleavage (Fig. 5.27), sometimes replaced by a horizontal tunnel reaching the meniscosynovial junction. They were situated in the middle segment but occasionally extended into either posterior or anterior segments. Superimposed on this basic combination of lesions, other variable ruptures can arise due to the general fragility of the structure.

viii. Lateral discoid meniscus

Very frequently this is complete, covering the whole of the tibial plateau (Fig. 5.28), yet does not cause any particular symptoms. It may be a chance discovery at arthroscopy, but symptoms may occur in certain circumstances. Rupture can produce a transverse or longitudinal bucket handle tear formation (Fig. 5.29). Diagnosis is frequently difficult because some longitudinal ruptures may be incomplete and not apparent on the superior surface of the meniscus; they can be situated very near the meniscosynovial junction, making exploration with a hook most awkward. In such cases, arthrography may offer a better means of diagnosis.

The discoid cystic meniscus may present as 'a pseudo-bucket-handle tear' (Fig. 5.30) because the thickening of the free border of the discoid meniscus, which is situated in the intercondylar notch, can be responsible for the appearance of a bucket handle in the intercondylar area associated with accompanying symptoms.

The meniscofemoral ligament of Wrisberg which joins the posterior horn of the lateral

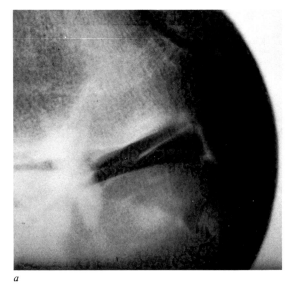

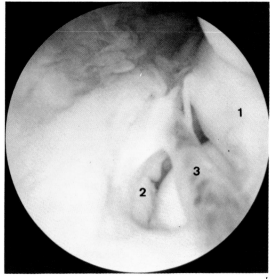

a

b

Figure 5.24. *Posterior detachment of the lateral meniscus. (a) Arthrography shows a very clear outline of the popliteal hiatus; (b) the arthroscopic appearance through a posterolateral approach: 1. the lateral meniscus; 2. the detached synovium; 3. a synovial bridge covering in part the posterior margin of the tibial plateau.*

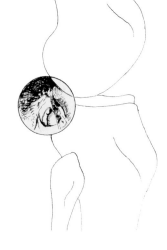

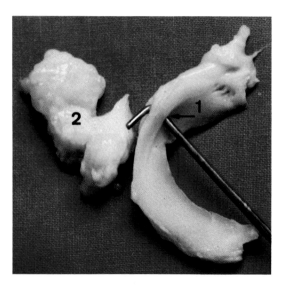

Figure 5.25. *Cyst of the lateral meniscus associated with a horizontal cleavage, sometimes represented by a simple tunnel (1), and a peripheral cyst of variable volume accessible by palpation (2).*

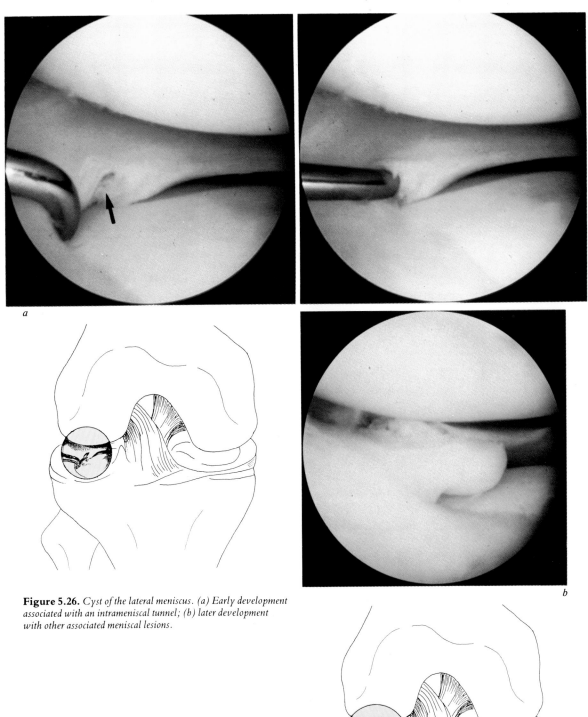

Figure 5.26. *Cyst of the lateral meniscus. (a) Early development associated with an intrameniscal tunnel; (b) later development with other associated meniscal lesions.*

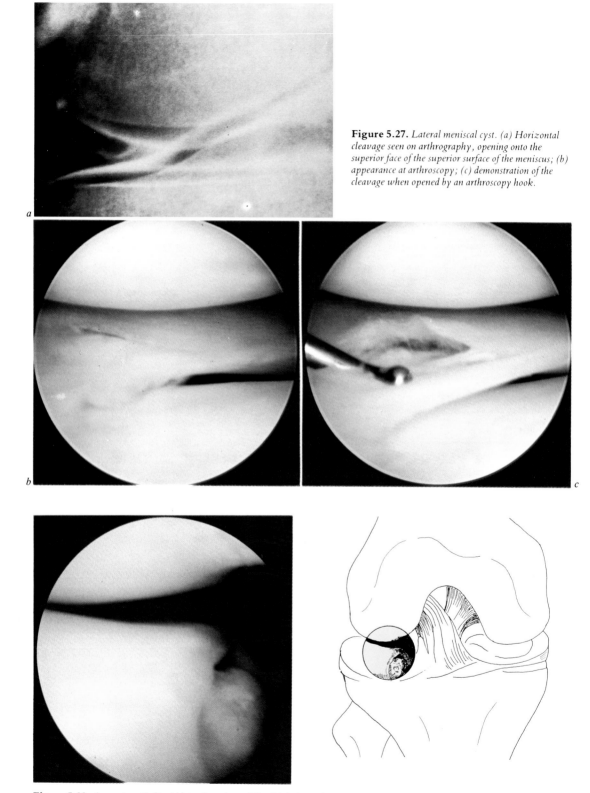

Figure 5.27. *Lateral meniscal cyst. (a) Horizontal cleavage seen on arthrography, opening onto the superior face of the superior surface of the meniscus; (b) appearance at arthroscopy; (c) demonstration of the cleavage when opened by an arthroscopy hook.*

Figure 5.28. *Asymptomatic discoid lateral meniscus. The tibial plateau is not seen.*

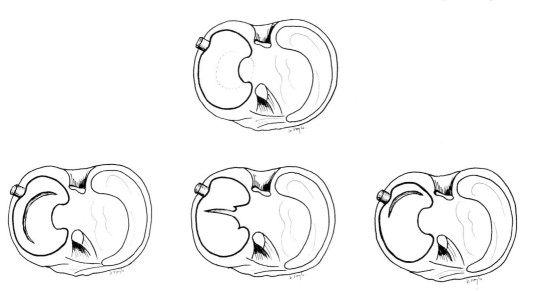

Figure 5.29. *Appearance of various ruptures of a lateral discoid meniscus.*

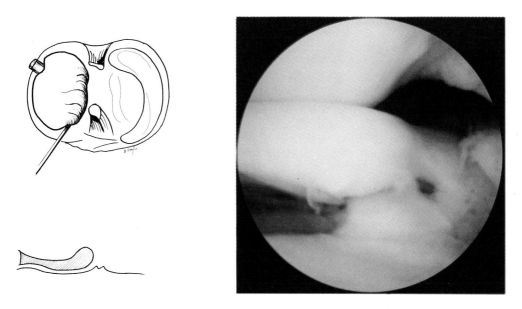

Figure 5.30. *Lateral discoid meniscus. The free border situated adjacent to the intercondylar space is thickened, giving an initial appearance of a displaced bucket handle tear.*

meniscus to the femur can be responsible, because of its shortness, for abnormal mobility of the lateral discoid meniscus during movements of flexion and extension. This hypermobility can cause posterior meniscal lesions.

General principles of arthroscopic meniscectomy

Arthroscopic surgery was not responsible for the change to concept of conservative meniscectomy from that of the original total menis-

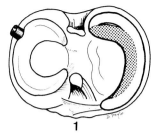 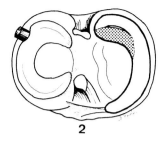

Figure 5.31. *Extent of meniscal resection. 1. During classic open operative procedure; 2. during arthroscopic meniscectomy when a partial resection is possible.*

cectomy. This shift was advocated in France by Albert Trillat with his concept of 'intramural meniscectomy'. Arthroscopy enables accurate diagnosis and surgery but should not, in our view, be regarded as a simple copy of meniscectomy by open arthrotomy; the important difference is that the close technique permits a partial meniscectomy in which it is not necessary, as it is the case with the open technique, to perform an intramural resection of variable extent towards the anterior segment (Fig. 5.31). Resection can be confined to the posterior segment.

Lanny Johnson stated that ideal, partial meniscectomy should remove abnormal and abnormally mobile meniscal tissue only. This concept is applicable to open and closed meniscectomy. Arthroscopy, however, gives a better appreciation of the quality of residual meniscal tissue, permitting economical and precise resection. Only if the *whole* meniscus is pathological should a total meniscectomy be performed.

The amount of meniscal resection depends upon a number of factors:

i. The extent of the lesion towards the periphery (this may be better evaluated by arthrography).
ii. The mobility of the meniscus as assessed by palpation with the arthroscopy hook, especially towards the end of the procedure when persistent cleavages of abnormal mobilities may be demonstrated and require further attention (Fig. 5.32). The mobility of the residual meniscus should also be tested by stopping the irrigation fluid and aspirating temporarily through the arthroscope so as to demonstrate any possible collapse of the residual tissue into

the joint space. The presence of moderate degrees of irregularity in the sectioned surface of the residual meniscal tissue is not of great importance because subsequent modelling will occur. However, the overall quality of the wall must be ensured. It is often useful to smooth it using the cutter. Finally, a simple technique offers a useful test of the residual meniscal tissue, that is, manual posteromedial or posterolateral compression at the level of the joint space which can propel any residual tissue into the tibiofemoral compartment under direct vision (Figs. 5.33 and 5.34).

The junction between the intact meniscus and the excised area must be sufficiently smoothed to avoid the possible formation of a subsequent tongue lesion (Fig. 5.35). It is imperative to avoid a loss of continuity between segments of residual meniscus, even if this is very narrow. Continuity of the meniscal rim is a mechanical factor controlling distension and gliding and it must be preserved (Fig. 5.36).

The quality of arthroscopic meniscectomy may be assessed on the appearance of the residual tissue as well as the state of the neighbouring articular cartilage. Avoidance of articular cartilage damage cannot be overemphasized. It is with experience, gentleness, quality of visual access, judicious choice of instruments, and, in particular, the opening of the tibiofemoral joint spaces that cartilage damage can be avoided. While the above and subsequent advice may be useful, only experience and practice will guide the individual operator to personalize the technique to best advantage.

Two main procedures are embodied in arthroscopic meniscectomy:

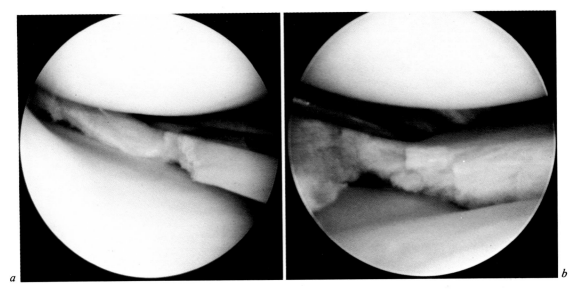

a   *b*

Figure 5.32. *Examination with an arthroscopy hook of residual meniscal wall, studying its mobility. (a) Medial meniscal wall; (b) lateral meniscal wall: the hook is introduced into the popliteal hiatus.*

●   Morselization, usually with the basket forceps, by means of which meniscal tissue is removed progressively in small fragments, these being liberated into the joint and subsequently removed regularly by irrigation.

●   Gross fragment excision separated by scissors or basket forceps; in general, this is a more elegant and rapid procedure and applicable especially to, for example, the removal of a bucket handle.

Arthroscopic surgery is usually conducted through two ports, anterolateral and anteromedial. One is for the arthroscope and the other for the operating instruments while both ports are interchangeable for these purposes.

Beware of losing a large fragment; this can be avoided by grasping it firmly so that it can be removed immediately after separation.

The utilization of three approaches is reserved for difficult situations; it is always inconvenient and cumbersome because of the small amount of space available, but does have the advantage of allowing meniscal section while exerting traction.

The choice of instruments is fundamental. The operator will quickly learn to make the right choice through experience and personal habit. We will not repeat the description of the instruments in detail, but merely remind the reader of certain concepts:

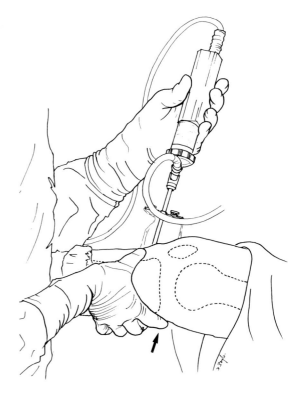

Figure 5.33. *Local manual pressure posteromedially in order to obtain optimal visual access to the posterior part of the medial meniscus.*

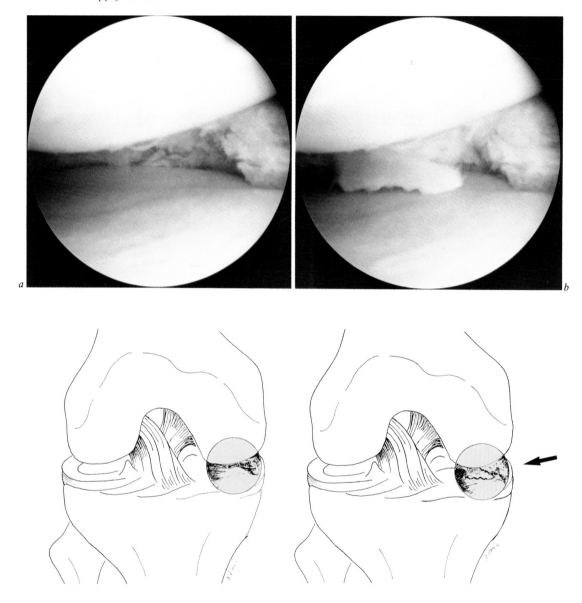

Figure 5.34. *Local manual pressure posteromedially. (a) The medial wall of the posterior segment after a local meniscal excision: the distension created by irrigation distends the wall which appears normal; (b) exteriorization by local posteromedial manual pressure of a large tongue which must be removed.*

(a)   The basket forceps, in our experience, has replaced the straight scissors: it allows morselization as well as section of a fragment of the meniscus. The direction of cut allows control of both the axis and extent.

(b)   Angulated scissors at 20° and 60° are indispensable for cutting the anterior part of the meniscus.

(c)   The meniscectomy knife is used very rarely. It must be used delicately because of the risk of using the tibial plateau as a cutting block.

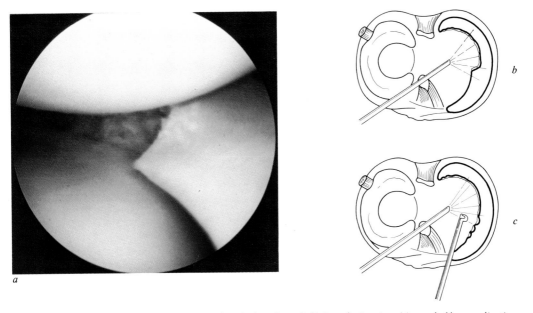

Figure 5.35. *Junction between excised meniscus and residual meniscus. (a,b) Irregular junction; (c) smoothed by morselization.*

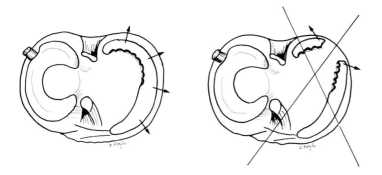

Figure 5.36. *Rupture of the continuity of the residual meniscal wall allows loss of resistance to circumferential distension.*

Medial meniscectomy

Positioning

It is preferable to place the arthroscopy stirrup with the tourniquet inflated fairly near to the knee. Throughout the procedure, the operator has to exert some degree of valgus stress to reach the posterior segment of the meniscus; it is important to ensure that the stressing does not translate to an internal rotation of the thigh (Fig. 5.37). This proximity of the support to the knee while useful is not indispensable. Experience shows that it is always possible to obtain valgus stressing satisfactorily, even with the tourniquet placed high, by lowering the operating table so as to avoid flexion of the knee.

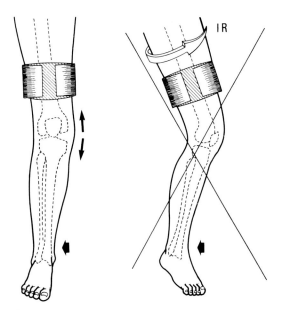

Figure 5.37. *Valgus stress allows opening of the medial tibiofemoral joint space. Internal rotation (IR) of the thigh must be avoided for this transforms the effect of the valgus to one of flexion of the knee.*

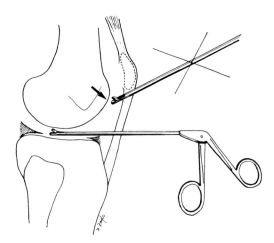

Figure 5.38. *A sufficiently low anteromedial approach allows direct access to the posterior segment of the meniscus, avoiding the convexity of the femoral condyle.*

Ports of entry

Uses of the anterolateral and anteromedial ports are sufficient in the majority of cases. We shall see later the rare indications for three approaches. Usually the arthroscope is introduced anterolaterally. Choice of the anteromedial port requires great care: it is necessary to be able to reach the posterior segment with ease (that being the commonest site of lesions of the medial meniscus) while avoiding the major obstacle, which is the internal condyle of the femur. Thus, the approach must be as low as possible, almost resting on the meniscus, in order to achieve a horizontal passage parallel to the tibial plateau (Fig. 5.38).

The arthroscope placed through the anterolateral port allows visualization of the anterior segment. A needle is introduced through the anteromedial aspect so that it is seen to enter the joint just above the medial meniscus with its direction parallel to the tibial surface. Once this site and direction is determined precisely, the needle is replaced by a knife carrying a number eleven blade having the same direction as the needle; again, under visual control, the positioning of the knife blade (which must not

damage the medial meniscus itself, nor the adjacent femoral articular cartilage) is confirmed. The orifice is then enlarged with forceps in order to permit passage of the instruments.

The tibiofemoral compartment is opened as widely as possible and after thorough evaluation of the lesion by palpation with the hook, surgery can proceed.

Techniques of medial meniscectomy

According to the type of meniscal lesion, the operator can plan the broad type of operative tactic necessary. We will outline these as follows:

i. Transverse rupture

The isolated transverse rupture situated at the free border is less common than that seen on the lateral side. Partial meniscectomy aims to regularize the free border of the meniscus so as to remove the rupture as far as it extends, and then to smooth the free border adjacently. At the end of this procedure, the hook is used to verify the quality of the excision and ensure that there is no horizontal component associated with the excised area left in the residual rim of the meniscus.

ii. Tongue lesion (parrot beak tear) (Fig. 5.39)

The treatment of tongue lesions constitutes one of the primary indications for operative arthroscopy, particularly in the posterior segment. The principle of management is simple and involves section of the base of the tongue with a knife or with scissors, or with the basket forceps, and then ablation with the forceps. An economic excision regularizing the residual margin of the meniscus is sometimes necessary both at its root and at the site of detachment. The discovery of a tongue with a pedicle directed anteriorly or posteriorly indicates the possibility of a bucket handle torn in its medial part, and the need to look for another tongue.

iii. Longitudinal lesion (Fig. 5.40)

This involves predominantly the posterior segment. When it is through the whole thickness of the meniscus, a sectioning of its posterior attachment is the first step, using, preferably, the basket forceps, or the scissors (Figs. 5.41 and 5.42). It is of advantage at this stage to smooth the posterior horn. The operator uses the hook to confirm that the posterior section is complete. Then the arthroscope and instruments are directed to the middle segment of the meniscus where the anterior attachment of the fragment is lifted. Here, a curvilinear section, harmonious with the zone of transition to the healthy meniscus must be achieved. It is not possible to modify the direction of the instruments, for their point of entry by the anteromedial port is fixed: it is therefore necessary to use angulated scissors of varying degrees to obtain a smoothly rounded cut. The instruments are held tangentially to the site of the cut required. Beginning with the 60° angulated scissors, the cut proceeds, and then the 20° angulated scissors are used so as to continue the section progressively in a direction corresponding to the anterior free margin. Finally, in order to complete the curvilinear line of section, straight basket forceps are used. The meniscal fragment is thus completely separated

and is best held by very fine traction forceps which grasp the end of the liberated fragment. As always, the meniscal residual wall is carefully inspected and palpated. Particular attention should be paid to the junction between the excised area and the residual healthy meniscus anteriorly. Sometimes some 'nibbling' with the 90° angulated basket forceps is necessary.

The longitudinal rupture in the posterior segment of the meniscus may be incomplete and perhaps only visible on the inferior surface of the meniscus. This may occur frequently and must not be missed. Treatment comprises a posterior section and then an anterior section; the latter must be extended progressively in the incomplete rupture of the meniscus and be completed with angulated scissors of varying degrees in order to follow exactly the direction of the fissure, which rejoins the posterior section performed first.

iv. Bucket handle tears (Figs. 5.43–5.45)

With practice, excision of a bucket handle tear is performed much more rapidly than is possible through an open arthrotomy. It is easily done using the anterolateral and anteromedial ports. Contrary to classic open surgery, the key to the intervention is first, the reduction of the bucket handle, if it is displaced into the intercondylar area, which allows section of its posterior end. The reduction is obtained by pressure with a hook on the bucket handle, associated with a sufficient opening of the femorotibial joint space by valgus stress. If the reduction is difficult—a rare occurrence—the hook may be replaced by meniscal forceps which can seize the anterior part of the bucket handle in order to exert a traction anteriorly and towards the peripheral wall.

Once reduction has been achieved, the situation becomes clear; the arthroscope, which is no longer impeded by the voluminous displaced meniscal fragment in the intercondylar area, can be passed freely through this space and the posterior end of the bucket handle can be sectioned accurately in the manner described above for the longitudinal rupture. As before, it is necessary to use the hook to check the quality of this section and that it is complete. The arthroscope is then lightly withdrawn and orientated towards the anterior end, which is

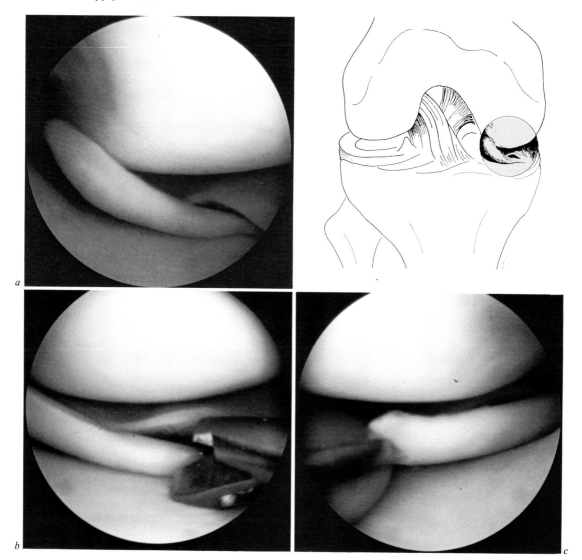

Figure 5.39. *Tongue or parrot beak tear of the medial meniscus. (a) The appearance of the tongue; (b) section of its pedicle by basket forceps; (c) extraction.*

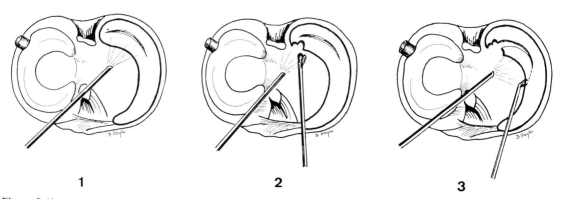

1   **2**   **3**

Figure 5.40. *Longitudinal rupture. 1. Exploration of the rupture; 2. section of the posterior attachment; 3. section of the anterior attachment.*

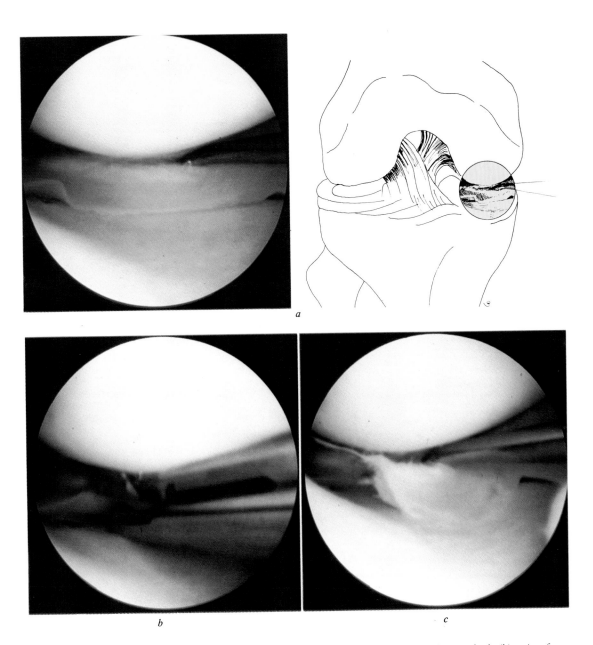

a

b   *c*

Figure 5.41. *Posterior longitudinal rupture. (a) Appearance of the rupture when explored with the arthroscopy hook; (b) section of the posterior attachment using basket forceps; (c) mobilization with the hook verifies that the section of the posterior attachment is complete.*

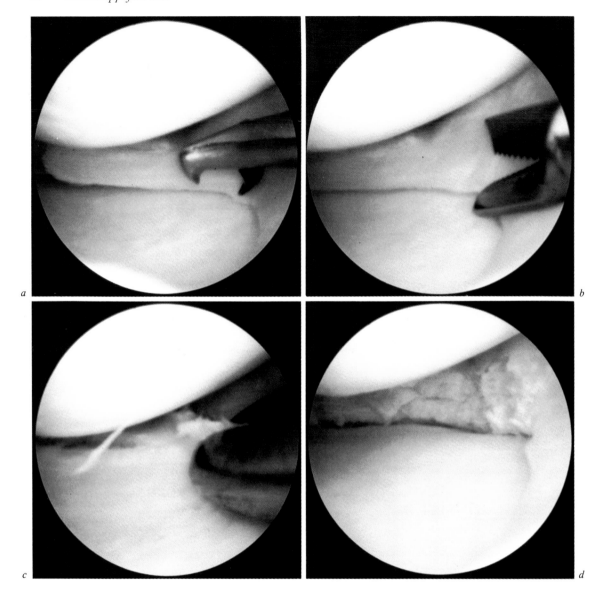

Figure 5.42. *Posterior longitudinal rupture (continued). (a,b) Section of the anterior attachment utilizing the 60° and then the 20° angulated scissors; (c) extraction of the fragment using forceps; (d) appearance of the residual meniscal wall at close of procedure.*

sectioned with 60° angulated scissors. Grasping forceps, or perhaps better the disc forceps, are applied to the anterior end of the bucket handle, and this allows extraction of the fragment. It is always necessary to ensure that the anteromedial port has been made sufficiently large for removal of the fragment, thereby avoiding hitching of the capsulosynovial tissue. It suffices to enlarge this orifice with forceps, having detached the meniscal segment. It is also preferable to grasp the detached fragment at its anterior end, rather than in its middle part, in

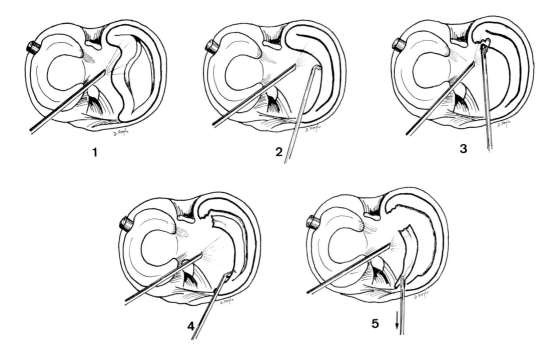

Figure 5.43. *Bucket handle tear of the medial meniscus: 1. bucket handle displaced into the intercondylar space; 2. reduction of the bucket handle; 3. section of its posterior attachment; 4. section of its anterior attachment; 5. removal.*

order to avoid difficulties in extraction due to folding.

Again, careful inspection of the residual meniscus must be conducted; it is not rare to find a double bucket handle which, again, must be excised totally.

The reason for beginning section of the bucket handle posteriorly is that if an anterior section is performed first, second section posteriorly becomes difficult because the meniscal fragment is no longer held anteriorly and tends to fold and relax during attempts at the posterior cut. Also, the liberated anterior fragment floats freely in the joint and can obscure the view through the arthroscope.

v. Meniscosynovial excision

If diagnosis indicates a detachment at the meniscosynovial junction, arthrography will provide the additional information as to the

type of lesion involved. It may be an occasion where a meniscal repair is preferable to excision. Repair is always better, especially considering our experience that there is frequently an accompanying rupture of the anterior cruciate ligament which also requires treatment. When arthrography indicates that suture is not appropriate, arthroscopic resection can be performed with the same technique as that used for posterior longitudinal ruptures, with the added factor that the excised fragment is much larger. It may be mentioned that arthroscopic suture is a possible technique, but at present it is too soon to judge the indications and its results.

vi. Degenerative meniscosis (Figs. 5.46–5.48)

This comprises complex lesions, which defy exact description, and which usually involve

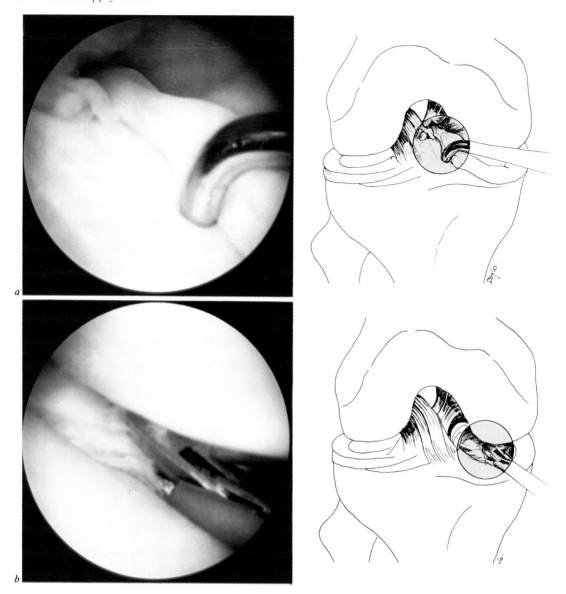

Figure 5.44. *Bucket handle tear of the medial meniscus (continued). (a) Reduction of the bucket handle previously displaced into the intercondylar area; (b) section of its posterior attachment using basket forceps.*

the posterior and middle segments. Longitudinal components are commonly associated with transverse components. Treatment is essentially that of morselization using the bucket forceps and perhaps the cutter. This last technique achieves a very economical regularization, a factor of prognostic importance because of the associated tibiofemoral arthrosis.

In spite of this, the possible need to realign the knee by osteotomy at a later stage must not be overlooked.

vii. Medial meniscal cyst (Fig. 5.49)

Rare in the medial meniscus, these tend to be

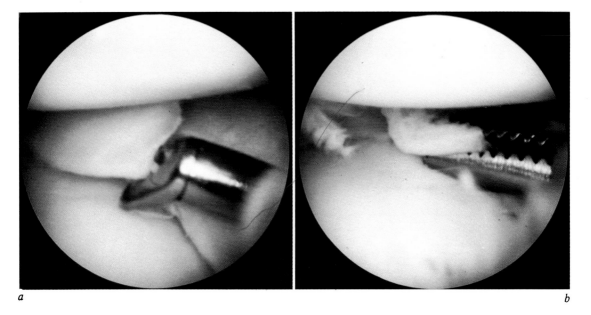

a   *b*

Figure 5.45. *Bucket handle of the medial meniscus (continued). (a) Division of anterior attachment using 60° angulated scissors; (b) grasping of anterior extremity using meniscus forceps.*

associated with a horizontal cleavage extending to the meniscosynovial junction. Therefore, meniscectomy has to be sufficiently extensive. It is possible to morselize progressively, although it is more elegant and rapid to remove the involved tissue by several broad cuts. The arthroscopic technique will be discussed further when considering the lateral meniscal cyst.

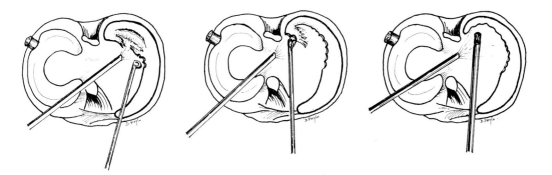

Figure 5.46. *Treatment of degenerative meniscosis using basket forceps and then the cutter.*

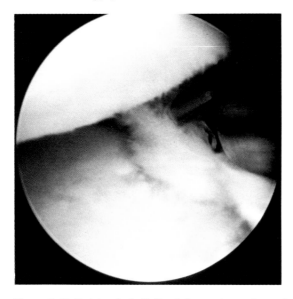
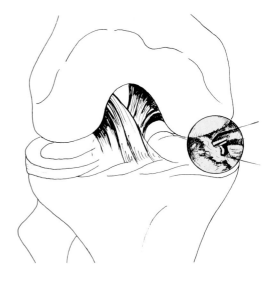

Figure 5.47. *Excision of soft, fibrillated, degenerative meniscus using the cutter.*

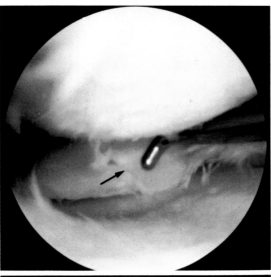
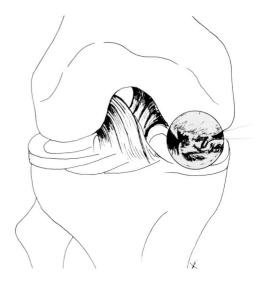

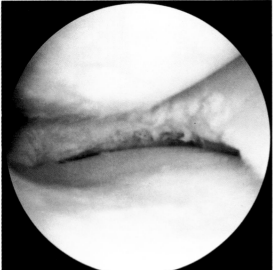

Figure 5.48. *Degenerative meniscosis with transverse rupture (indicated by arrow). Appearance at close of intervention with preservation of a good residual meniscal wall.*

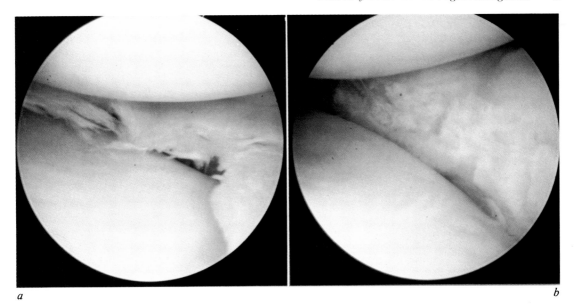

a   *b*

Figure 5.49. *Cyst of the medial meniscus. (a) Appearance of extended lesions; (b) after total arthroscopic resection.*

Lateral meniscectomy

Positioning

The support of the limb is as usual, with the stirrup placed near to the knee joint. Varus stressing is applied with the knee lightly flexed: a too marked degree of flexion actually impedes the effect of varus stressing as well as the circulation of the lavage fluid. As before, in order to avoid the rotatory effect of too much flexion, it is advisable to lower the table so that an appropriate angle can be achieved.

Ports of entry

While the anteromedial approach remains similar, the anterolateral port should be situated a little lower than usual, thus facilitating access to the posterior segment of the meniscus (Fig. 5.50).

Stressing varus causes a sliding of the cutaneous plane in relation to the capsule, and for this reason it is preferable to separate the site of antero-external puncture from the patellar

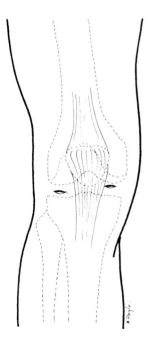

Figure 5.50. *Anterolateral and anteromedial approaches. The anterolateral approach is fairly low, in order to gain access to the posterior segment of the meniscus without being inconvenienced by the convexity of the femoral condyle. It is about 1 cm from the patellar tendon, allowing for sliding during varus stressing.*

tendon by 1 cm, in order to compensate for this relative sliding; this avoids bringing the cutaneous orifice over the tendon. Further, the separation of the capsular plane with respect to the cutaneous plane, produced by the varus stress, necessitates a second puncture with the scalpel through the same cutaneous orifice (Fig. 5.51). By this means, direct access to the meniscus is achieved, facilitating introduction of the instruments.

The use of two approaches ensures maximum efficiency in dealing with lateral meniscal lesions in terms of their site. Schematically (Fig. 5.52): the posterior and middle segments are more easily accessible to the instruments introduced through an anterolateral approach, while the arthroscope remains in the anteromedial port; for the anterior segment, access is easier by the anteromedial approach, using instruments angulated at 90°.

This arrangement is not always ideal and the operator should never hesitate to change the positions of the arthroscope and instruments according to need.

Particular features of the external meniscus

Certain peculiarities require a modification of the surgical technique on the lateral side:

- The physiological posterior mobility of the meniscus must be understood in order to appreciate its stability.
- Its thickness is much greater than that of the medial meniscus and may present particular difficulties in section, especially anteriorly.
- The presence of the popliteal hiatus modifies the strategy necessary in a resection of a meniscal bridge in relation to the popliteal hiatus, which is a significant factor in stabilizing the posterior segment. If this bridge is excised, the posterior segment may become excessively mobile and must then be excised. If the bridge can be partially conserved, the cohesion of the total ensemble of the meniscus will be better preserved and will allow conservation of the posterior segment. Moreover, the tendon of the popliteus is at significant risk during operative surgery, and it is absolutely essential to avoid any blind instrumental manoeuvre which could result in injury.
- Finally, the external meniscus is peculiar in its range of anatomical variations (for example, the discoid meniscus) and by its

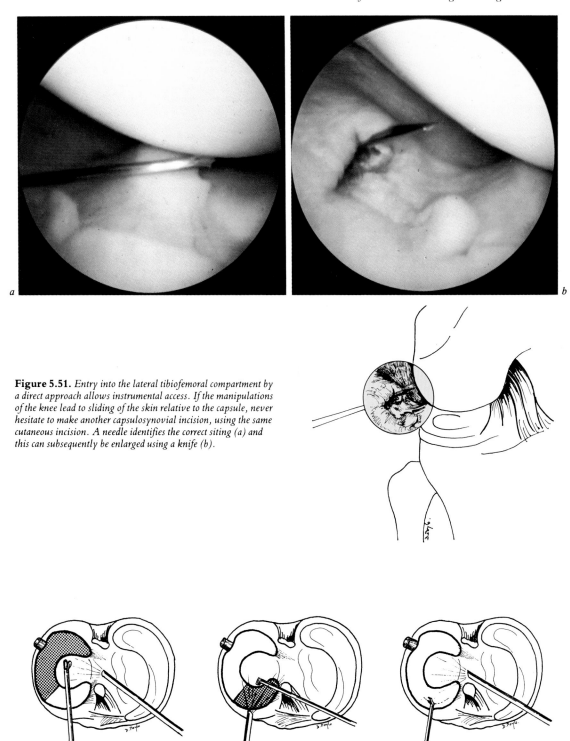

Figure 5.51. *Entry into the lateral tibiofemoral compartment by a direct approach allows instrumental access. If the manipulations of the knee lead to sliding of the skin relative to the capsule, never hesitate to make another capsulosynovial incision, using the same cutaneous incision. A needle identifies the correct siting (a) and this can subsequently be enlarged using a knife (b).*

Figure 5.52. *Possible uses of two approaches suitable for seeing and treating the lateral meniscus.*

involvement in cyst formation to which we shall return later.

Techniques of lateral meniscectomy

As with the medial meniscus, the therapeutic approach should be adapted to the type of lesion encountered:

i. Transverse rupture (Figs 5.53 and 5.54)

The excision necessitates the creation of a smooth border of the residual meniscus. The lesion is found most commonly in the middle segment and, at this site, the direction of the instrument is more or less tangential; the instrument of choice should therefore be angulated; for the direct excision of fragments, angulated scissors of variable degree are necessary. At the end of the excision, it is essential that the residual border should be smooth and taper progressively towards the margins of the intact meniscus. It is most important that a careful search for a possible cystic tunnel should be made at the end of the excision.

iii. Longitudinal rupture (Fig. 5.55)

When situated *posteriorly* (Fig. 5.56) the rupture should be followed along its course towards the posterior horn and then anteriorly, using scissors or basket forceps. The meniscal fragment is liberated. Sometimes, especially when the rupture is incomplete, progressive morselization is preferable. Careful assessment of the residual meniscus should be made in case there is a horizontal cleavage, and the quality of the stability of the meniscal bridge across the popliteal tendon should be assessed.

Anterior longitudinal ruptures are best approached using angulated scissors (Fig. 5.57) introduced through the anterolateral port. These cut through the entire thickness of the apex of the rupture, first posteriorly as far as the free border and then anteriorly, so as to liberate the meniscal fragment. Ninety degree angulated basket forceps or the cutter are most useful in regularizing the residual meniscal wall.

Whether the longitudinal rupture is anteriorly or posteriorly disposed, it is always preferable to commence the section directed towards

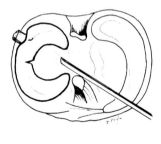 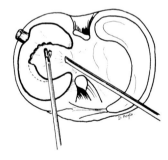

Figure 5.53. *Smoothing of a transverse rupture of the lateral meniscus.*

ii. Tongue lesion (parrot beak)

The pedicle of the parrot beak is sectioned and the tongue removed. The stump should be smooth and careful assessment of the quality of the residual meniscus made. Particular care should be taken not to lose the tongue and, therefore, before it is completely sectioned, extraction forceps should be applied.

the posterior end. If the anterior part is released first, the liberated tongue of meniscal tissue is likely to obscure the arthroscopic view.

iv. Bucket handle tear (Figs. 5.58–5.60)

The technique of excision is similar to that for the medial meniscus—reduction of the bucket

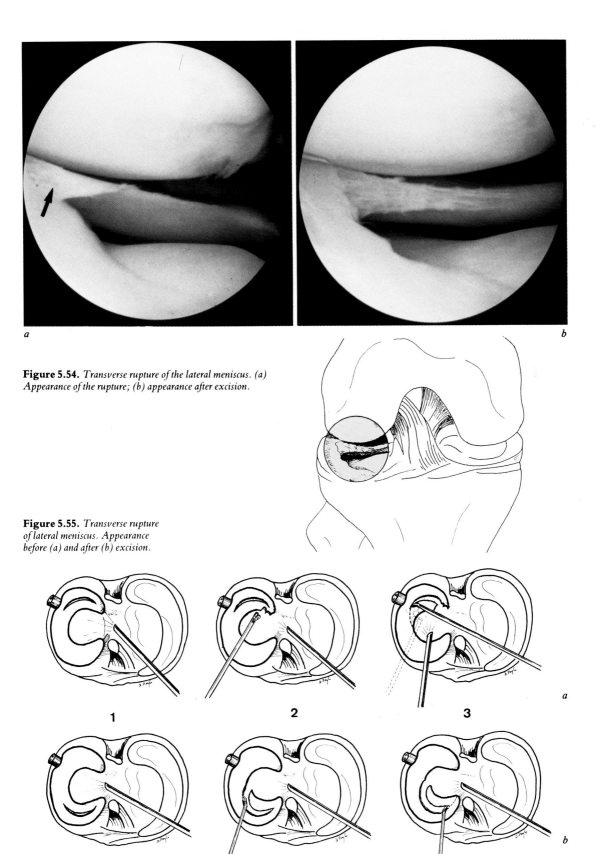

Figure 5.54. *Transverse rupture of the lateral meniscus. (a) Appearance of the rupture; (b) appearance after excision.*

Figure 5.55. *Transverse rupture of lateral meniscus. Appearance before (a) and after (b) excision.*

1 2 3

a

b

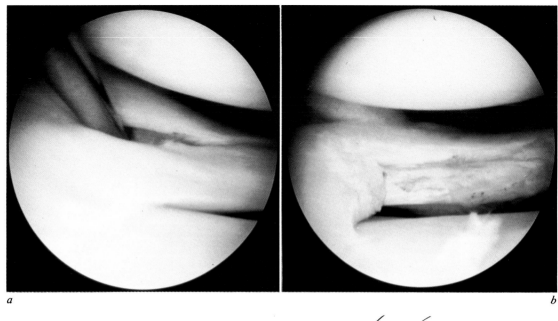

a   *b*

Figure 5.56. *(a) Posterior longitudinal rupture of the lateral meniscus; (b) appearance after meniscal excision. Note the importance of conserving an adequate meniscal bridge across the popliteal hiatus.*

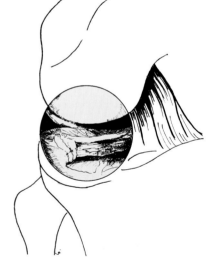

handle, division of its posterior attachment with the basket forceps, division of the anterior attachment with the 60° angulated scissors, and then extraction using traction forceps.

Particular difficulties relate to the, occasionally, large volume of the bucket handle, especially in cases associated with a lateral discoid meniscus. Sometimes, the reduction itself may be impossible, necessitating division of the bucket handle inside the intercondylar

area. In such circumstances, the operator should not hesitate to use a third port of entry in order to insert traction forceps to the meniscus so as to facilitate its posterior section.

v. Posterior meniscosynovial detachment

The meniscosynovial rupture should be sutured whenever possible. We perform this procedure

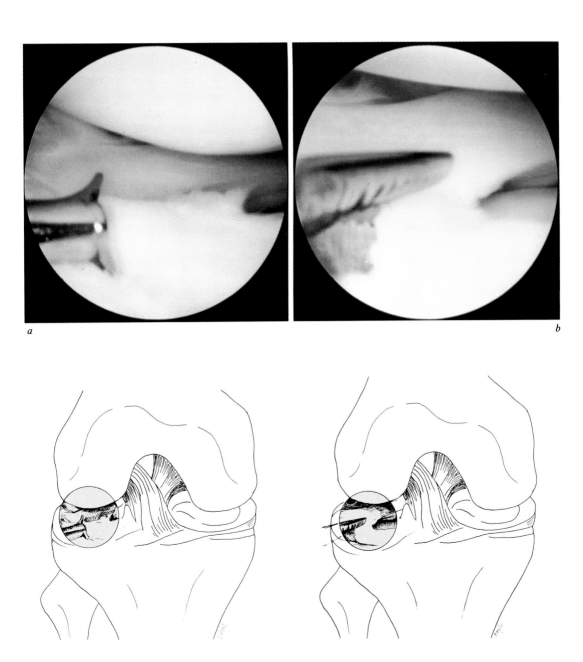

Figure 5.57. *Anterior longitudinal rupture. Use of the 60° (a) and then 20° (b) angulated scissors allows section of the meniscus progressively towards its free border.*

as an open posterolateral operation. If repair is not possible, the whole posterior segment, including the popliteal meniscal bridge, must be removed and tapered anteriorly in the middle segment, the anterior segment being entirely undisturbed.

vi. Degenerative meniscosis

Excision of all loose tissue leaving a sufficiently stable residual meniscal wall can be best achieved using the cutter.

vii. Lateral meniscal cyst

The aim of operative arthroscopy is twofold: the excision of all pathological meniscal tissue and saucerization of the cyst by widely opening it into the joint or, better, by excision of the walls of the cyst.

While classic surgical treatment by arthrotomy has necessitated a total meniscectomy, arthroscopic resection allows a conservative procedure in which the anterior and posterior segments can usually be preserved undisturbed. At the middle segment, the excision must follow as far as the periphery at the site of the cyst, but with conservation of a narrow bridge of meniscal tissue joining the posterior and anterior segments which will contribute to the stability of the whole remaining meniscal ensemble.

Operative technique is as follows (Fig. 5.61): (a) partial excision of the anterior segment following on to the middle segment utilizing the 60° angulated scissors introduced through the anterolateral port, followed by (b) partial excision of the posterior segment progressing

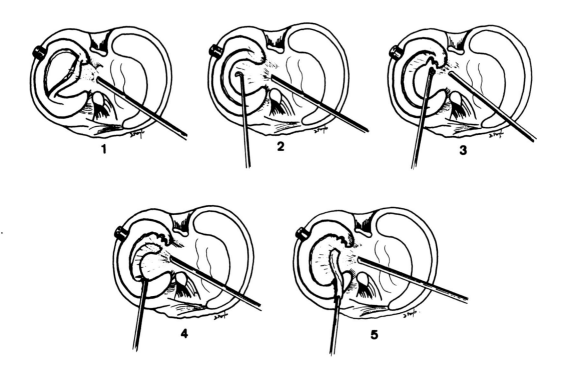

Figure 5.58. *Stages in the management of a bucket handle tear: 1. the appearance of the displaced bucket handle; 2. reduction using a hook; 3. section of posterior attachment; 4. section of anterior attachment; 5. extraction.*

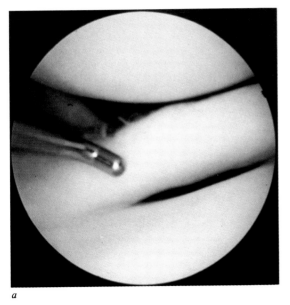

a

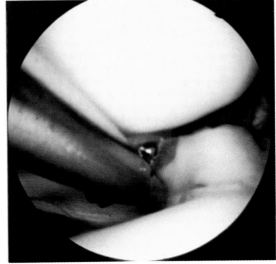

b

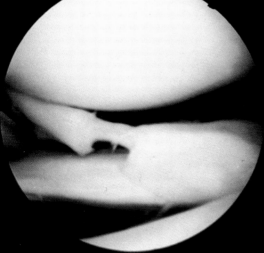

c

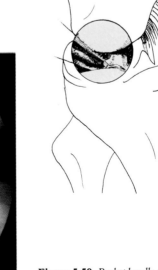

Figure 5.59. *Bucket handle of lateral meniscus: (a) bucket handle displaced and reduced using hook; (b) section of posterior attachment using basket forceps; (c) verification of posterior section—in this view it is incomplete.*

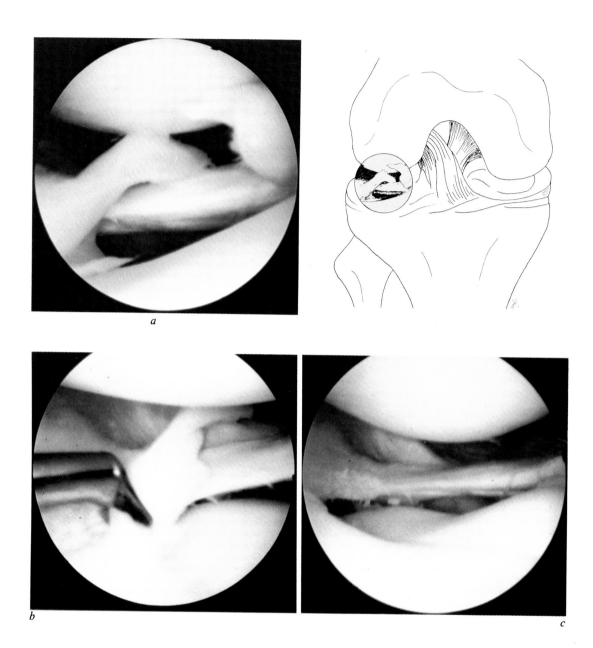

Figure 5.60. *Bucket handle tear of lateral meniscus (continued): (a) posterior section is now complete; (b) anterior section; (c) appearance of residual meniscal wall at close of procedure.*

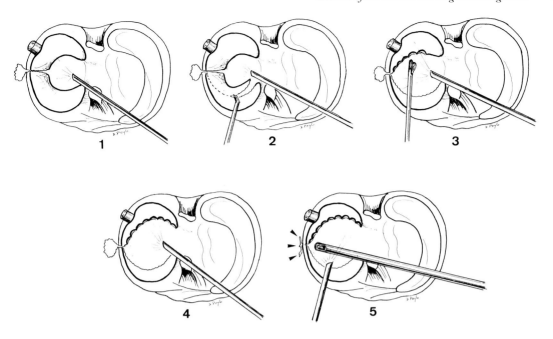

Figure 5.61. *Technique of treatment of cyst of the lateral meniscus: 1. the appearance; 2. excision of the middle and anterior parts; 3. excision of the posterior part; 4. appearance of the residual meniscal wall conserved; 5. excision of the cyst periphery using the cutter.*

forward, by morselization, into the middle segment using the basket forceps. (c) The excision of these two segments is conducted progressively towards the middle segment in such a manner that the periphery of the meniscus is approached near the site of the cyst (there may be a tunnel or a cleavage). A slender bridge of meniscal tissue should be preserved at the site of the cyst. Similarly, the meniscal bridge at the site of the popliteal hiatus can usually be preserved, but in some instances it may be necessary, because of extension of the meniscal lesion into this area, to excise totally the posterior segment if it becomes too mobile. (d) The excision of the walls of the cyst (Fig. 5.62) completes the meniscectomy. The instrument of choice is the cutter and it is introduced into the cyst usually through the anteromedial approach. Its cutting and aspirating action allows a progressive removal of the cyst. If a cutter is not available, it is necessary to eventrate the cyst by means of basket forceps so that the area communicates widely with the joint.

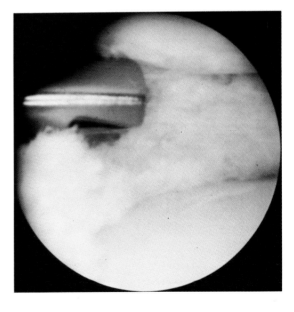

Figure 5.62. *Excision of the peripheral part of cyst using cutter.*

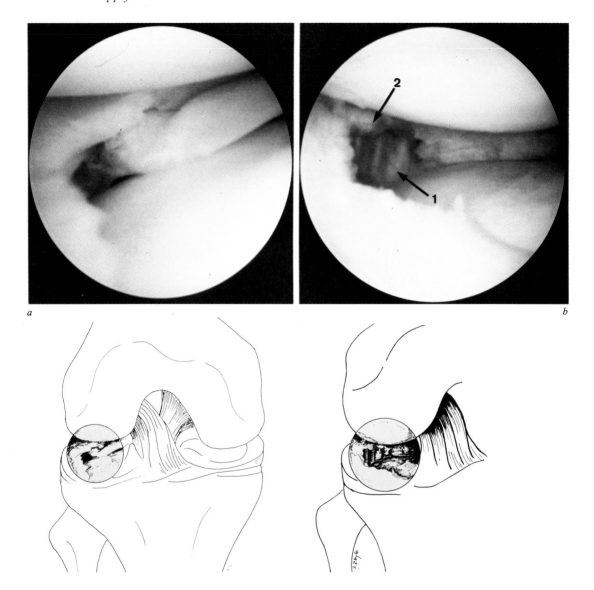

Figure 5.63. *Cyst of the lateral meniscus: (a) appearance of the lesion; (b) residual meniscal wall at close of intervention. Excision of the wall of the cyst reveals the fascialata (1). A small bridge of meniscal tissue is preserved (2).*

It is perfectly possible, using the anteromedial and anterolateral approaches, to effect a partial meniscectomy, completed by the flattening and obliteration of the cyst (Figs 5.63–5.66).

viii. Lateral discoid meniscus

When necessary, excision of a lateral discoid meniscus is possible by arthroscopic surgery (Fig. 5.67); however, this procedure can be difficult. The technique depends on the experience of the operator and the difficulties encountered, but the aim is to remove the bulk of the meniscus, leaving a meniscal wall of similar size to that of a normal meniscus (Fig. 5.68).

A transverse section of the central area using angulated scissors leaves the free border at an appropriate distance from the periphery so as to leave a normal size meniscal wall. The anterior

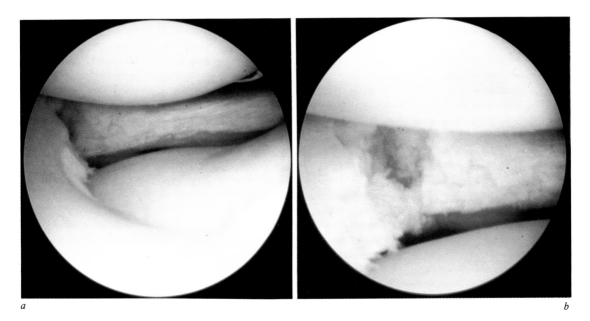

a   *b*

Figure 5.64. *Cyst of the lateral meniscus. Appearance of the residual wall after excision. (a) Anterior and posterior segments are preserved; (b) the cystic pouch has been excised. There remains a small inferior meniscal bridge joining the anterior and posterior segments.*

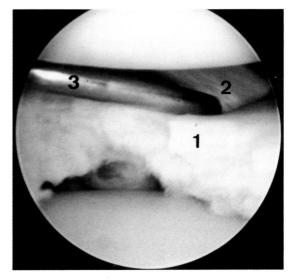

Figure 5.65. *Appearance at end of excision of meniscal cyst testing stability of the residual meniscal bridge (1) in relation to the popliteal tendon (2) by traction with the hook (3).*

section using the angulated scissors rejoins the free border towards the front. The section then proceeds posteriorly. Thus, it is possible to detach and separate a large anterior fragment. This allows the final stage of excision of the posterior segment, maybe using the scissors or, perhaps, by morselization. The free border of the meniscal wall should be finally regularized using the cutter leaving in place a meniscus with a normal appearance.

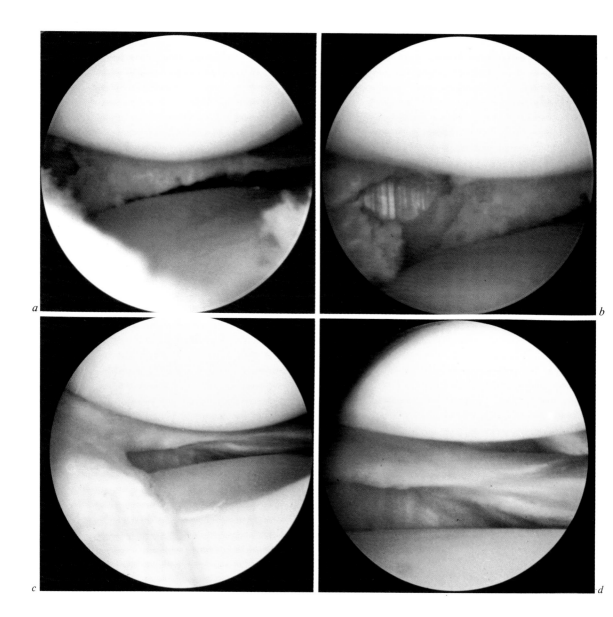

Figure 5.66. *Cyst of the lateral meniscus: (a,b) appearance at close of procedure. The cystic pouch, excised, is situated just in front of the popliteal hiatus; (c,d) appearance later, the meniscal wall having become smoothed and regenerated at the margins of the original cyst.*

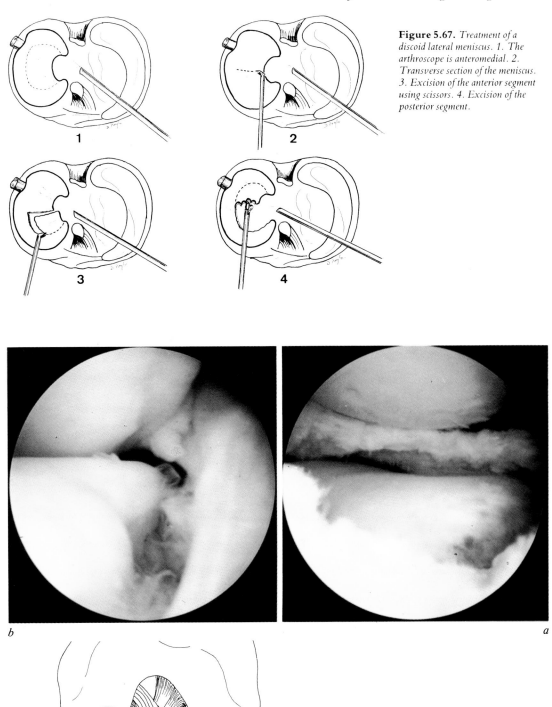

Figure 5.67. *Treatment of a discoid lateral meniscus. 1. The arthroscope is anteromedial. 2. Transverse section of the meniscus. 3. Excision of the anterior segment using scissors. 4. Excision of the posterior segment.*

Figure 5.68. *(a) Discoid lateral meniscus with free thickened border; (b) after excision.*

Difficult meniscectomies

While all meniscal lesions *can* in theory be excised by arthroscopic surgery, there are cases which require all the operator's skill and experience. The major risk is that of damage to the articular cartilage. It is always best to foresee the difficulties and, if the procedure is problematic, prudently resort to arthrotomy: this is better than damaging the joint surfaces! With experience the operator will need to resort to open arthrotomy less and less frequently.

Particular difficulties relate to the type of meniscal lesion, difficulties of visual access, especially to the posterior segment, as well as instrumental access to the same area.

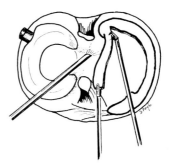

Figure 5.69. *Three ports of entry are used for the ablation of a difficult bucket handle tear.*

1. Difficulty related to the anatomical type of meniscal lesion

Removal of the bucket handle of the medial meniscus can be difficult if it is irreducible, if it is already detached anteriorly so that it floats and obscures vision or, if after the usual first section of the posterior end followed by detachment of the anterior end, it is found that the posterior detachment was not complete. In these circumstances, we advise the use of three ports of entry (Fig. 5.69): the anterolateral one for the arthroscope, and two anteromedial ports, one enlarged in order to allow easy removal of the possibly bulky bucket handle by means of meniscal grasping forceps, which can gain firm purchase on the anterior end of the bucket handle. Traction must be exerted, so that the structure is firmly held, while through the second anteromedial puncture, another instrument, most commonly straight basket forceps, can be inserted so as to detach the posterior part of the bucket handle. The traction exerted by the grasping forceps facilitates work on the posterior part even as far back as the posterior horn. Three ports are not commonly required, but should be used readily when indicated.

Another difficulty can occur when the tongue of a tear in the posterior compartment displaces into the back of the posteromedial area (Fig. 5.70); it is easy to miss such a situation. The simplest solution is certainly to manipulate the fragment using an arthroscopy hook; it may be necessary for the arthroscope to cross the intercondylar area in order to perform this manoeuvre under direct vision.

2. Difficulties relating to access to the posterior meniscal segment

Difficulty can occur when the available space between the femoral and tibial surfaces is small due to the knee being tight despite effective valgus and varus stressing.

More subtly, a rupture of the anterior cruciate ligament may make the opening of the joint space difficult, particularly on the medial

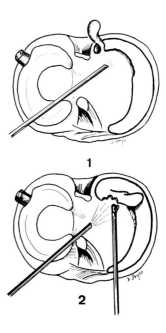

Figure 5.70. *1. Posterior parrot beak tilted into the posteromedial compartment. 2. Section after reduction to the medial tibiofemoral compartment.*

side; valgus stressing with the knee a little flexed produces, in effect, a Lachman manoeuvre, with the opening of the tibiofemoral space being replaced by a sliding of the tibial plateaux anteriorly, amounting to a tibial subluxation. This can preclude all access to the posterior segments of the menisci. The situation may be improved by maintaining the leg in external rotation when exerting the valgus stress.

In cases where posterior access is difficult, the risk to the articular surface is significantly increased. It is necessary to have sufficiently small instruments available and to introduce them gently into the meagre tibiofemoral space. Even small instruments, during their backwards and forwards manipulation, can damage the surfaces. The cutter is particularly useful in these circumstances because it is only necessary to place the operating end in position on one occasion.

Manual pressure over the posteromedial and posterolateral aspects of the knee joint can aid visualization of the posterior meniscal segments very usefully. The posterior meniscal segments can be pushed forward directly into the joint space and therefore become more accessible.

3. Visualization difficulties from other causes

These include synovial hypertrophy, chondral fibrillation, and complex meniscal lesions sometimes with hypertrophy and ragged, stringy degeneration. Visual access to both anterior and posterior ends may be impossible and preclude all possibility of excision. It is in these difficult cases that the shaver is invaluable, in that it allows a general cleaning of the tissue: with this instrument, synovial excision, smoothing of ragged articular surface of the condyles, and primary trimming of the meniscus are all possible. The intervention can then proceed in conditions of much better visual access.

The above descriptions are only guidelines which must be adapted according to the type of meniscal excision necessary. A strategy, based on what is to be expected from the outset, always offers the best chance of a smooth successful intervention.

6

Synovial membrane

Henri Dorfmann*

The state of the synovial membrane is affected by any articular cartilage disorder, exceptionally at the juxta-articular margin, or it may be the primary site of disease. Arthroscopy allows direct assessment of its appearance and facilitates biopsy if necessary. Technically, the procedure has no special feature, except perhaps the more frequent use of local anaesthesia when the synovium is the only structure likely to be examined; the superolateral port is more frequently used and it is better not to use a tourniquet, because normal vascularization may be used to interpret certain images.

The *indications* for synovial arthroscopy relate primarily to the diagnosis of a mono-arthropathy of uncertain origin. It is unusual for the procedure to be necessary in the case of a polyarthritis.

Normal synovial membrane

In most areas this is smooth, transparent, and marked by fine blood vessels. In various zones, according to the type of joint, fine translucent villous formations present and these usually contain a central vessel.

In the knee the normal villi locate on the floor of the suprapatellar pouch (Fig. 6.1). Sometimes these can be fatty and enlarged, with a yellowish hue, but are still normal (Fig. 6.2). The latter should be distinguished from true fatty hypertrophy which can accompany, in particular, some arthroses.

*Department of Rheumatology, Centre Hospitalier, 93602 Aulnay-sous-Bois, France.

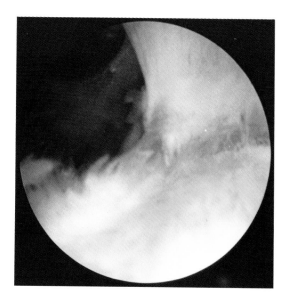

Figure 6.1. *Opening of the suprapatellar pouch showing the appearance of normal synovial membrane of the floor.*

Mechanical synovitis

This term implies a synovial reaction to some mechanical disorder of the joint, the synovium itself not being the primary site of disease. It is characterized by a modification of the villi. These lose their transparency and become partially or totally opaque; their number may be increased, but overall they conserve a normal villus form; often, they appear somewhat stocky, and have been described as resembling short grass (Fig. 6.3).

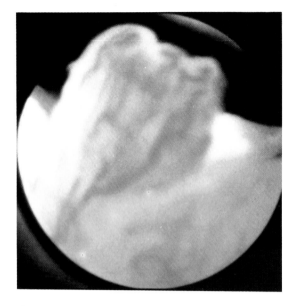

Figure 6.2. *Fatty synovium.*

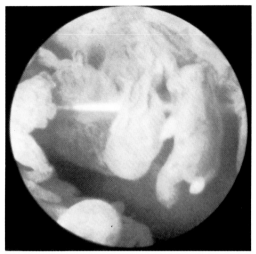

Figure 6.4. *Proliferative inflammatory synovitis.*

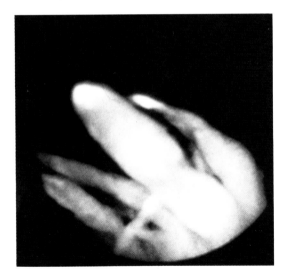

Figure 6.3. *Mechanical synovitis.*

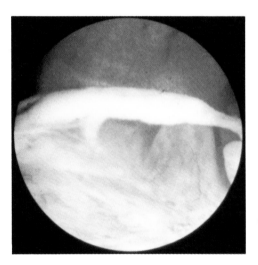

Figure 6.5. *Bridge of fibrin.*

Inflammatory synovitis

The appearance of inflammatory synovitis is very different (Fig. 6.4). In agreement with Watanabe[1] we have distinguished four types. It is the massive proliferation of large villi which characterizes an inflammatory synovitis, and which usually makes it easy to distinguish this from mechanical synovitis. The proliferative type includes two subgroups of which the more common is characterized by noticeable oedema, whereas less commonly there is a synovial proliferation associated with the release of fibrin (Fig. 6.5). In contrast, the synovial membrane may be smooth, oedematous and hyperaemic, or may appear sclerosed (Figs. 6.6 and 6.7). These four types of appearance usually correspond well with the histological

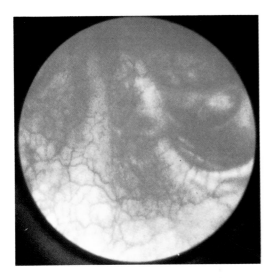

Figure 6.6. *Appearance of oedematous and hyperaemic synovium.*

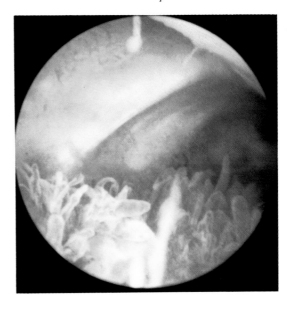

Figure 6.8. *Proliferative synovitis of an intermediate degree.*

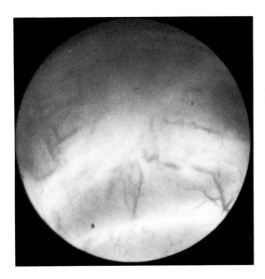

Figure 6.7. *Sclerosed synovium.*

findings. The proliferative type especially has always been thus confirmed[2] but the smooth type of synovitis must be taken into consideration with both clinical and histological findings.

While typical examples of mechanical and inflammatory synovitis are easy to distinguish, there exist threshold cases (Fig. 6.8) in which the synovial membrane presents with numerous opaque folded villi which nevertheless maintain overall a normal shape. These can be due to an early evolving inflammatory condition, or a resolving one, or perhaps to an exceptionally violent mechanical response. In all instances, biopsy and histological study are necessary.

We have sought to identify the specific appearances of the synovium in rheumatoid arthritis in which there exist large ridges of fibrin or, especially, pannus formation (Fig. 6.9), and the particular features favouring a diagnosis of tuberculosis (Fig. 6.10).[3] With experience, these conditions can be distinguished but must always be confirmed by biopsy and the general clinical picture.

An exceptional finding may be the discovery of a synovial metastasis.[4]

The conditions described below, although much less common, are much more easily recognized by direct observation of the synovium.

Chondromatosis

In its typical form, diagnosis is often made by the discovery and evacuation of dozens or even hundreds of small lentil-shaped cartilagenous

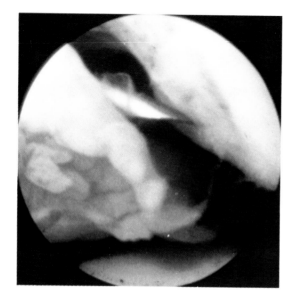

Figure 6.9. *Rheumatoid pannus.*

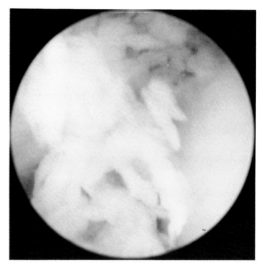

Figure 6.11. *Agglutinated masses of chondroma.*

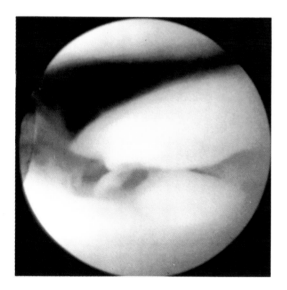

Figure 6.10. *Tuberculous synovitis.*

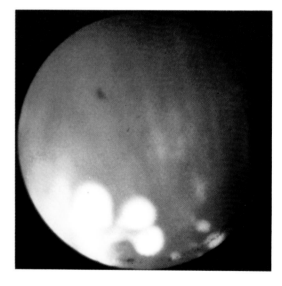

Figure 6.12. *Pedunculated chondromata on the synovium.*

fragments. On other occasions, it is in one part of the joint that the bodies of various size sometimes adhere together like bunches of grapes. They can be evacuated by lavage (Fig. 6.11). With regard to the appearance of the synovial membrane, in some instances it may appear normal while in others it presents with numerous folded villi forming small globules on the summits of which may be observed cartilagenous bodies; sometimes these are attached by fine pedicles (Fig. 6.12). The histology biopsy specimen in typical form exhibits cartilagenous intra-synovial meta-plasia.[5]

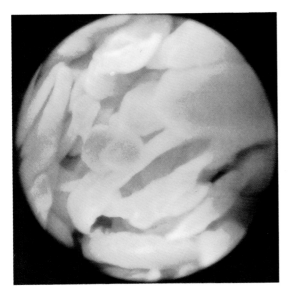

Figure 6.13. *Appearance of villonodular synovitis.*

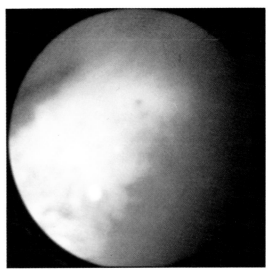

Figure 6.15. *Microcrystalline masses.*

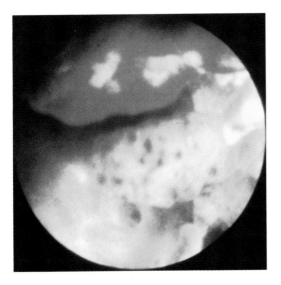

Figure 6.14. *Pseudopurpuric synovitis in a villonodular condition under tourniquet.*

Pigmented villonodular synovitis

The isolated *pseudotumoral nodular* form is always extra-articular but Beguin *et al.*[6] have reported six cases (and we ourselves have had one case) in which the lesion in the knee has been intra-articular. The usual symptoms from these have been essentially mechanical, related to the size of the swelling produced. At arthroscopy, the tumour may be of variable size and of flabby consistency or, more frequently, pedunculated with vascular appearance.

The more usual manifestation of the disease is of a *diffuse form* occupying all or part of the articular cavity. Profuse elongated villus proliferation, fine and characteristically brownish, may be the predominant appearance, but sometimes these may include nodular formations with small rounded swellings (Fig. 6.13). The essential characteristic, whether villous or nodular, is the brownish colouration and the proliferation of the synovium. When arthroscopy is conducted with the tourniquet applied, the nodules characteristically have areas of violet staining after exsanguination, resembling a pseudopurpura (Fig. 6.14).

Crystal arthropathy

The depots of microcrystals, usually calcium based but sometimes urate, are easily recognized as pinhead-sized incrustations over the whole synovial surface (Fig. 6.15). Their appearance on the synovial membrane is, in our experience, much less common than on the adjacent articular cartilage and menisci.

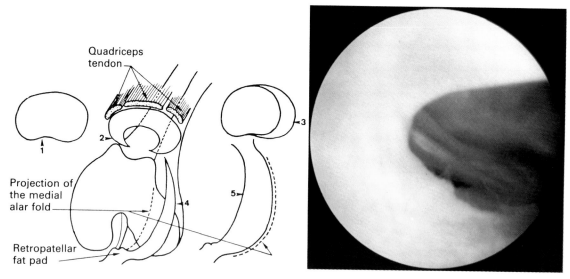

Figure 6.16. *Various presentations of synovial plicae: 1–3 superior; 4, 5 medial.*

Figure 6.17. *Medial end of superior plica.*

Filarial arthritis

In modern life, the occurrence of filarial infestation is no longer a rarity. If the diagnosis is suspected from eosinophilia in the joint fluid and especially the presence of microfilariae, arthroscopy may sometimes allow identification of the adult filaria in the joint.[7]

Synovial reduplication—plica

Synovial reduplication constitutes a pathology specific to the knee and strongly merits recognition. It is necessary to appreciate the anatomy in order to understand the pathological effects produced by these synovial folds which are formed by the permanent adhesion of two adjacent layers of synovial membrane. According to their site, they may be identified as superior, inferior, and medial. They are easily visible at arthroscopy (Fig. 6.16).

i. Superior synovial plica

This is a remnant of the membrane which in the embryo separates the subquadricipital bursa from the main joint cavity. In 10–13 per cent of cases, according to different authors, normal dehiscence does not occur, and a permanent septum persists; otherwise it is more or less complete leaving a central orifice of variable extent. More commonly, as a result of asymmetrical disappearance of the septum, there remains a medial remnant forming an arch-shaped strut, concave laterally (Fig. 6.17). Finally, the fold totally obliterates, but it is fairly easy always to recognize its site, there remaining a change in the appearance around the junction between the original true joint cavity and the suprapatellar pouch into which the arthroscope has been introduced. The frequency of recognition of the plica is variously reported, but I am of the opinion that this relates to the method of exploration and the attention paid to the area. It *is* important to understand that the plica, when the knee is extended, locates in a plane perpendicular to the axis of the femur extending from the anterior surface towards the posterior aspect of the quadriceps tendon, describing an arciform trajectory and terminating a little below the inferior pole of the patella; during flexion to 90°, its axis becomes progressively more parallel to the axis of the femur.

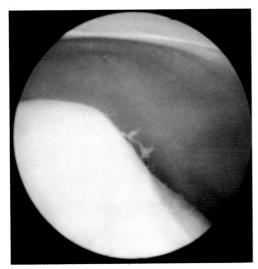

Figure 6.18. *Type 1 medial plica.*

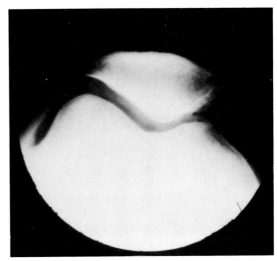

Figure 6.20. *Arthrogram, axial view, showing the alar fold above a medial plica.*

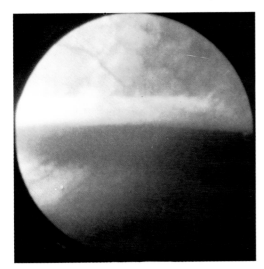

Figure 6.19. *Type 2 medial plica.*

ii. Medial synovial plica (synovial shelf)

The origin of this structure is debatable, but it is situated always on the medial wall of the joint cavity from which it obtrudes perpendicularly and, with the knee in extension, it lies parallel with the axis of the femur. There are three principle types: *Type 1* (Fig. 6.18) comprises a simple transverse extension of the medial part of the retropatellar fat pad. This may be easily missed unless it is sought systematically, particularly through a superior port and, accordingly, this probably accounts for the variability in the incidence of this lesion described in the literature. *Type 2* is the commoner variety (Fig. 6.19) and is the typical 'shelf' described in the English literature. It extends sideways from the patella fat pad and forms a little shelf-like structure separating upper and lower parts of the medial synovial wall. The synovial membrane is thin, vascularized and supple, and its position with respect to the intercondylar margin varies according to the degree of flexion of the knee. *Type 3* is much less common. It comprises a broad membrane extending above towards the superior plica described earlier which it may reach, covering the third facet of the patella, sometimes extending even to the medial facet margin, and always hooking across the condylar margin of the femoral condyle. Two sources of confusion exist: the medial plica should not be confused with the alar fold which is situated inferiorly (Fig. 6.20). The latter is related to the patella from which it descends outwards and inwards and comprises a simple draping of the synovial membrane elevated by vertical prolongations of the retropatellar fat pad. The second source of error relates to the fact that the medial plica can sometimes reach the site of remnant of the superior plica described earlier. There is confusion in the literature.[8-10] The medial remnant of the superior plica and the medial plica should be regarded as two different and independent structures.

iii. The inferior plica

This runs approximately parallel to the anterior cruciate ligament and from the upper limit of the retropatellar fat pad; it is directed towards the intercondylar notch, a little less obliquely and laterally than the cruciate ligament. Its development is variable, but on occasions can amount to a true septum impeding communication between the medial and lateral tibiofemoral compartments of the knee joint.

Interest in these plica has been stimulated by arthroscopic observation, which can now afford a true pathological entity.

In my view, it is the medial plica which has proved of clinical importance.[11] In the majority of cases, it produces symptoms typically in a young sporting subject, these supervening after trauma or microtrauma such as may result from a change in training technique. The typical sign is of an almost constant pain over the anteromedial aspect, sometimes occurring when squatting, which may be impossible. It can cause a sensation of instability or pseudolocking. The presence of a click may be experienced. Often the individual experiences a sensation of distension in the knee. Physical examination may detect the medial plica as a hypertrophied band rolling under the finger over the medial side of the knee a little inward of the medial border of the patella. A fixed point of tenderness a little above the joint line may be found. Sometimes, pain is experienced during flexion at about 60°. Less characteristic is the presence of an effusion or signs of patellofemoral pain. If the plica is visible at arthrography, then arthroscopy can be performed electively and may show the thick, avascular fibrous band (Fig. 6.21) which is seen to impinge against the trochlear or the condyle according to the degree of flexion. In the absence of treatment, there is a risk of producing a secondary chondropathy of the articular surface of the patella or of the trochlear area.

Symptoms arising from a superior plica are much less frequent, and indeed there is doubt as to whether they arise at all; certainly they have been much less described. Pain is sited near as for the medial meniscus, but at a higher level, above the patella. Pain does not occur at 30° but during flexion above 90°. The symptoms produced are probably related to a simple traction effect from the patella, the superior plica restraining movement of the knee—rather

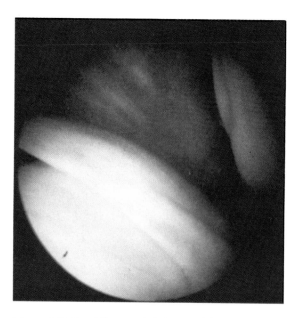

Figure 6.21. *Broad fibrous medial plica regarded as pathological. Note the abnormal articular cartilage of the patella opposite.*

than this being caused by an entrapment or direct impingement against the trochlear of the femoral condyle—which is responsible for the pain associated with a medial plica. However, it is possible that beyond 90° flexion, some degree of direct impingement could be involved. At arthroscopy, it is more difficult to prove the pathological nature of a superior fibrous plica, since even the normal superior plica is slightly vascular. It is only by the correspondence of clinical symptomatology and the absolute absence of any other pathological entity, together with the observation of a frankly fibrous nature of the plica, that a diagnosis can be accepted. In some 2500 arthroscopies, I have seen only twelve cases in which a superior plica has caused symptoms.

Until recently the inferior plica was considered completely innocuous. Courroy and Paclet have reported cases of traumatic rupture in young subjects with a haemarthrosis following trauma involving this plica.

Arthroscopic surgical management

Arthroscopic management contributes significantly to a variety of the synovial conditions mentioned above.

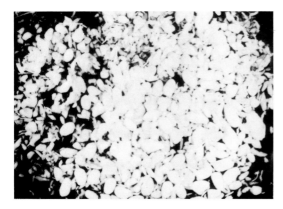

Figure 6.22. *Lavage of rice grain form bodies from polyarthritis.*

Articular lavage has been recommended for a number of conditions including several synovitides (Fig. 6.22). This procedure has in fact been practised in a blind fashion without arthroscopy under the name arthroclysis. O'Connor[12] has recommended it for chondrocalcinosis.

The procedure can amount to a true debridement of the joint cavity in chondromatosis including extraction (Fig. 6.23) or aspiration of all of the foreign bodies; excision of depots of fibrin found in rheumatoid synovitis may be performed, or in the case of filarial monoarthritis, extraction of the filarial and removal of fibrinous depots may be accomplished.

With the availability of motorized instruments, it is technically possible to perform partial or total synovectomy. In France, the latter has become less frequently practised unless accompanying some other procedure at open surgery. In contrast, partial synovectomy by arthroscopic means can be very useful in several rarer conditions, in particular, villonodular synovitis and localized chondromatosis.

Arthroscopy constitutes the treatment of choice for the synovial plica; complete excision (Fig. 6.24) is easily achieved. Statistics indicate a success rate of some 70–100 per cent, provided that the pathology is strictly isolated. Results are naturally poorer if the primary condition has resulted in chondropathy.

Arthroscopy methods have been advocated for division of post-operative or post-infective adhesions, thereby improving the effects of manipulation under general anaesthesia.[13] Such

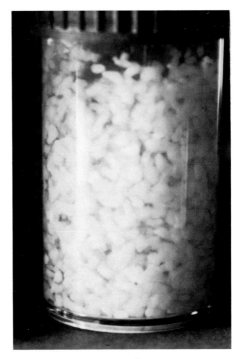

Figure 6.23. *Foreign bodies resulting from chondromatosis.*

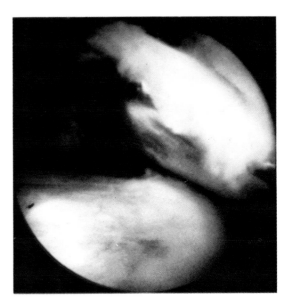

Figure 6.24. *Medial plica during resection using forceps.*

management is more effective if performed early. Adhesions can be located more readily in the suprapatellar pouch and collateral recesses. More recently, it has been recognized that the patellar retinacula can be resected.

References

1 Watanabe M, Takeda S, Ikeuchi H, *Atlas of arthroscopy* (3rd Ed. Tokyo, Igaku-Shoin Ed., 1978, 1 vol, 156 p).

2 Dorfmann H, Figueroa M, Sèze S De, 'Intérêt de l'arthroscopie devant une mono-arthropathie isolée due genou', *Sem Hop Paris* (1974) **50:** 179–188.

3 Dorfmann H, Dreyfus P, Justin-Besançon L, Sèze S De, 'Arthroscopie du genou. État actuel de la question', *Sem Hôp Paris* (1970) **46:** 3442–3450.

4 Guyader Souquières G, Mora JJ, Béguin J, 'Découverte arthroscopique d'une métastase synoviale révélatrice d'un adénocarcinome', *J Med Lyon* (April 1983) **1378:** 35–38.

5 Dorfmann H, D'Harcourt G, Bonvarlet JP, Boyer TH, 'Chondromatose du genou', *J Med Lyon* (Dec 1984) **1394:** 5–11.

6 Beguin J, Locker B, Souquières G, 'Tumeurs bénignes localisées de la synoviale du genou et arthroscopie—A propos de 6 cas', *J Med Lyon* (Feb 1984) **1386:** 25–28.

7 Dorfmann H, Sèze S De, 'Monoarthrites filariennes—A propos d'un cas diagnostiqué par arthroscopie', *Nouv Presse Med* (1972) **1:** 1013–1016

8 Hardacker WT, Whipple TL, Basset FH, 'Diagnostic and treatment of the plica syndrome of the knee', *J Bone Joint Surg* (1980) **62[A]:** 221–225.

9 Hughston JC, Whatley GS, Dodelin RA, Stone MM, 'The role of the suprapatellar plica in internal derangement of the knee', *Am J Orthop* (1963) **5:** 25–27.

10 Pipkin G, 'Lesion of the suprapatellar plica', *J Bone Joint Surg* (1950) **32[A]:** 363–369.

11 Dorfmann H, Orengo PH, Amarenco G, 'Pathologie des replis synoviaux du genou—Intérêt de l'arthroscopie', *Rev Rhum* (1982) **49(1):** 67–73.

12 O'Connor RL, *Arthroscopy* (JB Lippincott. Philadelphia, 1977, 1 vol, 173 p).

13 Sprague NF, O'Connor RL, Fox JM, 'Arthroscopic treatment of postoperative knee fibroarthrosis, *Clin Orthop* (1982) **166:** 165–172.

7

The ligaments

Consideration of the ligamentous structure of the knee ligaments relates almost entirely to the cruciate ligaments. Arthroscopy has a place in the diagnosis of recent and of old ruptures as well as in their treatment, but must be preceded by appropriate clinical examination and radiology.

The anterior cruciate ligament

Recent rupture

This may appear at arthroscopy as an interstitial haematoma (Fig. 7.1); a partial rupture affecting predominantly either the anteromedial or

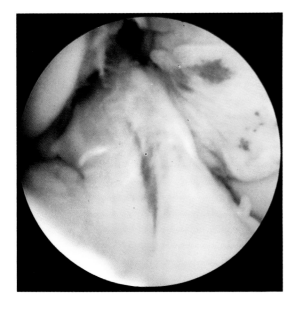

Figure 7.1. *Haematoma in the sheath of the anterior cruciate ligament.*

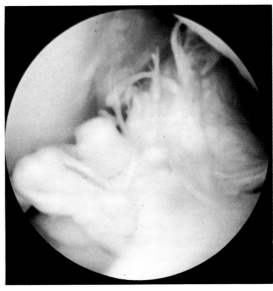

Figure 7.2. *Complete rupture of the anterior cruciate ligament.*

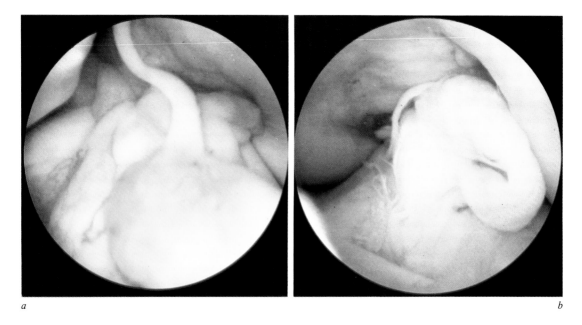

a   b

Figure 7.3. *Appearance of old ruptures of the anterior cruciate ligament. (a) Disappearance of the ligament with persistence of a synovial remnant; (b) ruptured ligament bunched at the level of its tibial attachment.*

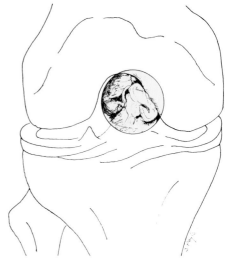

posterolateral fasciculi; or a total rupture in which the synovial sheath may or may not be intact (Fig. 7.2). The site of lesion is variable but frequently high, near to the femoral attachment.

Old rupture

Arthroscopic diagnosis may be easy but is sometimes difficult (Figs 7.3 and 7.4). The lesion is easily identified if the ligament has disappeared from the intercondylar area and the arthroscope approaches the posterior cruciate ligament directly. The ligament remnant may lie horizontally against the posterior cruciate ligament or it may present like the clapper of a bell, its free extremity become piriform as a result of repeated entrapment between either medial or lateral tibiofemoral joint components. This mechanical derangement can lead to a clinical diagnosis of a meniscal lesion.

Diagnosis may be difficult when the ligament remains in the intercondylar notch, visualization being impeded by synovial hypertrophy which must be excised. Diagnosis will then

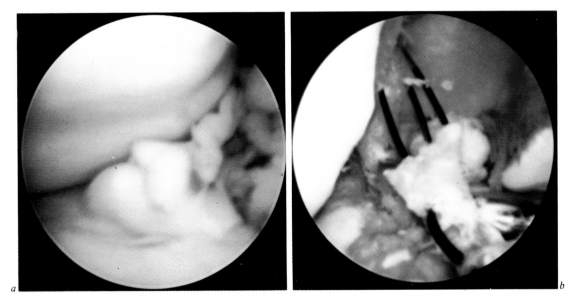

Figure 7.4. *Old rupture of the anterior cruciate ligament. (a) Appearance of a bell clapper interposed between the lateral femorotibial joint surfaces; (b) failure of a primary suture.*

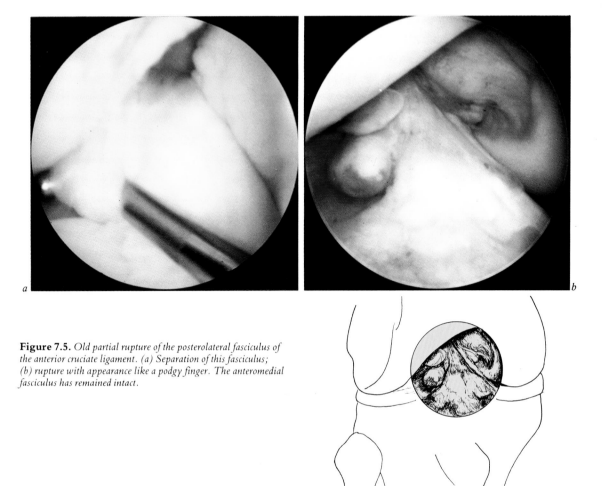

Figure 7.5. *Old partial rupture of the posterolateral fasciculus of the anterior cruciate ligament. (a) Separation of this fasciculus; (b) rupture with appearance like a podgy finger. The anteromedial fasciculus has remained intact.*

depend upon the appearance of the ligament after the excision, perhaps its horizontal direction, a precise study of the two fasciculae (Fig. 7.5) and, in particular, of their superior insertions; finally, tension of the ligament can be demonstrated using an arthroscopy hook. It should be clearly confirmed that the ligament tightens during internal rotation, during the anterior drawer test, and when valgus stress is exerted.

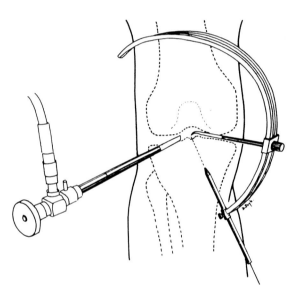

Operative arthroscopy

Techniques are continuously developing and various therapeutic possibilities exist.

(a)   Excision of residual ruptured anterior cruciate ligament, especially the entrapped bell clapper type.

(b)   Screwing of an avulsed tibial spine, which we have achieved on several occasions.

(c)   Femoral reattachment by stapling after freshening of the zone of implantation (Lanny Johnson).

(d)   Most significantly, ligamentoplasty using an autograft (patellar tendon, or one of the pes anserinus tendons) or by synthetic prosthesis. These ligamentous placements under arthroscopy are facilitated by using an appropriate jig (Fig. 7.6) which enables precise location of the necessary bony tunnels.

The posterior cruciate ligament

The anterior diagnostic approach is insufficient. It is necessary to introduce the arthroscope into the posterior compartment traversing the intercondylar notch, and to put the end of the instrument very near to the posterior cruciate ligament in order to obtain adequate vision. The posteromedial port is preferable and an arthroscopy hook should also be introduced.

Figure 7.6. *Ligamentoplasty of the anterior cruciate ligament by arthroscopy. (Above) Transtibial drill guide installed. The arthroscope permits ideal positioning of the guide inside the joint at the upper border of the tibia. The jig guides the drill to make a transtibial tunnel. (Right) Tunnel through the lateral femoral condyle after arthroscopic localization of the femoral attachment of the anterior cruciate ligament.*

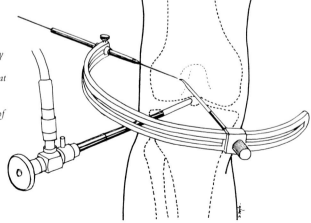

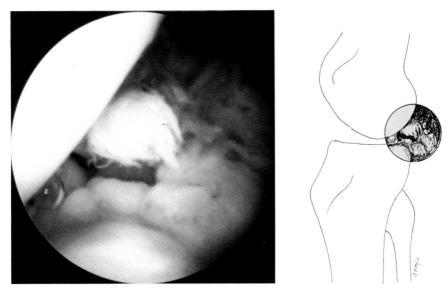

Figure 7.7. *Complete recent rupture of the posterior cruciate ligament seen through posteromedial port.*

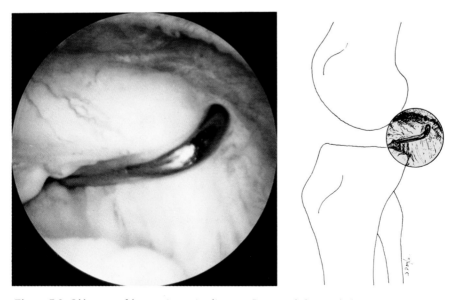

Figure 7.8. *Old rupture of the posterior cruciate ligament. Posteromedial port. The hook, introduced through the intercondylar notch, demonstrates the ligament separation.*

Recent rupture may appear complete (Fig. 7.7), interstitial (perhaps with a breach of the synovial sheath), or as a haematoma, indicating the site of a low or a high rupture near an attachment.

Old ruptures. As is the case for the anterior cruciate ligament injuries, arthroscopic diagnosis can sometimes be difficult, especially when the posterior cruciate ligament apparently maintains its proper orientation. It is essential to study its tension by palpation with the arthroscopy hook (Fig. 7.8), assess whether the tibia drops back with respect to the femur, and,

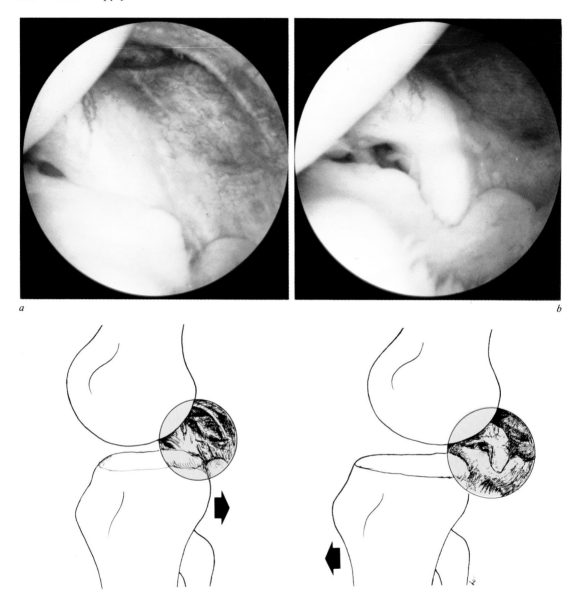

Figure 7.9. *Old rupture of the posterior cruciate ligament. Posteromedial approach. (a) The tibia is in its posterior drawer position; (b) on reduction of the posterior displacement, the posterior cruciate ligament becomes relaxed, but still preserves an angulated appearance, confirming its laxity.*

during the posterior drawer test, perhaps demonstrate separation of the ruptured area of the ligament (Fig. 7.9).

Ligamentous laxity

Diagnosis

Clinical and radiological examination have first priority. It is unusual for the clinical assessment not to detect rupture of the anterior or posterior cruciate ligaments (a jump on medial rotation of the tibia described by Lemaire, the Lachman sign, as well as anterior and posterior drawer augmentations). Plain radiology may demonstrate an avulsed bony fragment commonly at the tibial spine region, while arthrography can reveal a rupture of the anterior cruciate ligament, as well as demonstrating the integrity of the menisci.

Arthroscopy is rarely necessary to establish the diagnosis, but it does give further information which may be helpful, especially in the case of old lesions. Apart from direct observation of the cruciate structures themselves, the state of the menisci and of the articular surfaces can be verified, and, in particular, the condition of the femoral condyles may be of prognostic importance. Arthroscopy is contraindicated in severe sprains of the medial and lateral collateral ligaments because of the risk of further stretching by the lavage fluid pressure.

Treatment

Cruciate reconstructions have been mentioned earlier. For laxity problems with a positive instability jerk sign, the extra-articular ligamentoplasty arthroscopic technique described by Lemaire is preferable to open arthrotomy, in that it allows a precise treatment of the intra-articular lesions, economic resection of menisci, excision of a ruptured fragment of an anterior cruciate ligament, and articular cartilage shaving.

Arthroscopic surveillance

Arthroscopy is useful in following up the condition of intra-articular transplants, as well as in assessing the continued state of the menisci and the articular surfaces.

8

The articular surfaces

Osteocartilagenous abnormalities are frequent in the knee, and the diagnostic and therapeutic problems they pose are often complex. Arthroscopy has much to offer, although sufficiently long term follow-up of the techniques is not yet available to us for a complete assessment and their descriptions in this chapter are not intended to give the impression that they supplant classic orthopaedic operations of known value, such as valgus osteotomy and realignment of the patellar apparatus.

Osteoarthrosis

We have adopted the Ficat classification, which seems to us to correspond to arthroscopic observations. Like him, we can distinguish two evolving stages: a progressive chondrosis, followed by an osteoarthrosis, in which bony changes become apparent. The two stages are significantly different by virtue of their appearances and their therapeutic incidences.

Chondrosis

The condition is entirely confined to the articular cartilage and there is no bony involvement. Diagnosis may be difficult, since radiographs appear normal. It is here that arthroscopy can clarify the situation by a precise appraisal of the cartilagenous lesion and of its topography. According to Ficat the severity of the condition may be classified as follows:

Stage one: oedematous surface identifiable by palpation with the arthroscopy hook (Fig. 8.1).

Stage two: fissuring with tiny scaling of the articular cartilage, ulceration not reaching the subchondral area.

Stage three: subchondral involvement, where the deep tissue becomes partly exposed (Fig. 8.2).

Outside stage three, the thickness of the articular cartilage is difficult to assess during arthroscopy; a needle can be used to test the depth of cartilage under visual control.

Site

On the *patella* surface, stage one is frequent but its appreciation with the arthroscopy hook is a delicate manoeuvre because of the natural resilience of the articular cartilage at this site and also the effect of magnification of the arthroscopic image. It is necessary to palpate minutely the whole surface of the patella and to identify those zones which are clearly abnormally soft, by which means an accurate map of the medial and lateral articular facets and of the crest can be drawn.

An appreciation of the congruence of the patellofemoral articulation and of its stability is important, although again difficult to assess. A tilting or misalignment of the kneecap laterally, visible on patellofemoral radiographs, may be very clearly demonstrated at arthroscopy (Fig. 8.3) but, in contrast, evaluation of slight instabilities is difficult in the absence of precise criteria whatever the port of entry of the arthroscope, inferior or superior. Moreover, many factors considerably modify the appearance of the patellofemoral congruence; in

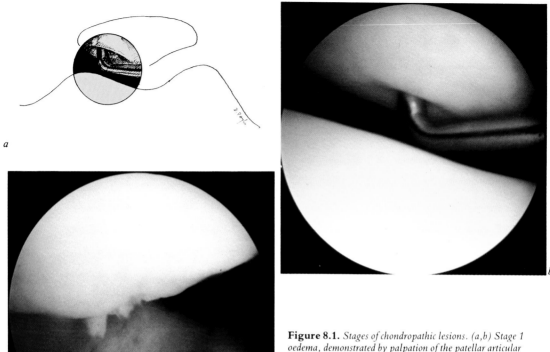

a

b

c

Figure 8.1. *Stages of chondropathic lesions. (a,b) Stage 1 oedema, demonstrated by palpation of the patellar articular surface; (c) stage 2 fissurization of the patellar articular surface.*

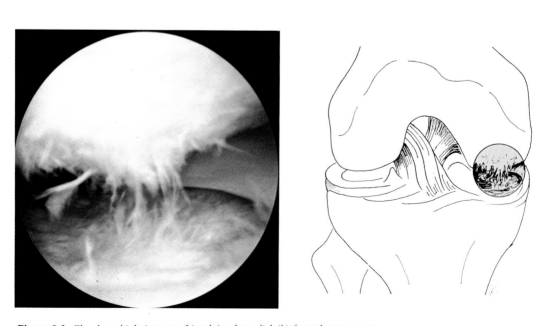

Figure 8.2. *Chondropathic lesions stage 3 involving the medial tibiofemoral compartment.*

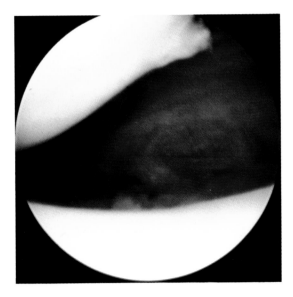

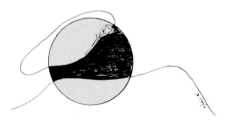

Figure 8.3. *Study of the congruence of the patellofemoral joint surfaces at 45° flexion of the knee. There exists in this case a significant tilting of the patella, with lateral subluxation.*

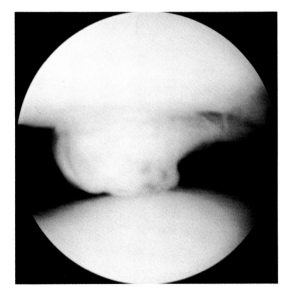

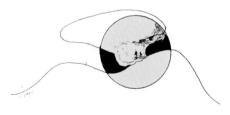

Figure 8.4. *Hypertrophic articular cartilage of the patella with protruberance.*

particular, the proximity of the tourniquet to the knee itself and the degree of articular distension by the lavage fluid, etc.

The *femoral trochlear surface* can exhibit sites of cartilagenous involvement on the shoulders and neck. These often relate to corresponding lesions on the patella. They may, however, be isolated and localized to the femoral aspect and be responsible for symptoms. The arthroscopy hook must be used assiduously with this in mind.

On the *femoral condyles*, cartilagenous involvement most frequently spares the anterior part, but develops to varying extents posteriorly. Its assessment necessitates sufficient flexion to unroll and expose the condyle adequately. Similarly, with the *tibial plateaux*, the posterior part related to the posterior segment of the menisci is the commoner site for development of osteoarthritis.

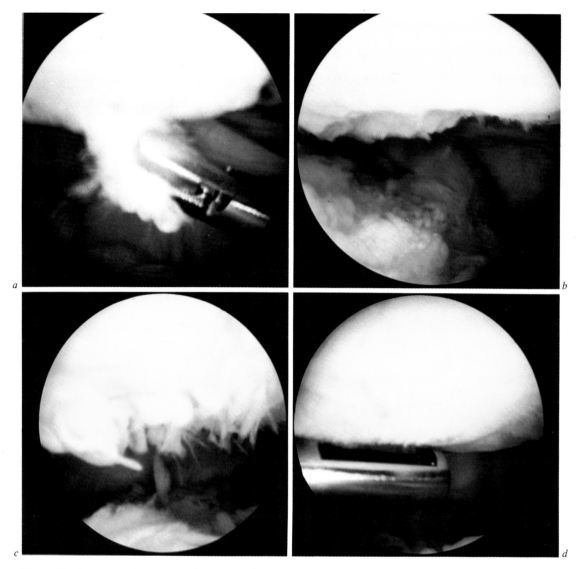

Figure 8.5. *Shaving articular cartilage surface of the patella (a,b) using the basket forceps, which excises tongues of cartilage transforming the lesion into a cartilagenous crater with regular borders; (c,d) using the shaver, the instrument of choice for a fibrillated chondropathy.*

Arthroscopic treatment

Essentially, treatment involves 'shaving' the cartilagenous surface, thereby smoothing it; the advantages are, firstly, the excision of projecting hypertrophic zones which have proliferated, producing cartilagenous masses which impinge between moving surfaces (most commonly around the patella) and, secondly, the excision of pathological cartilage transforming such areas into craters lined with smooth borders (Fig. 8.4).

Shaving is performed using the basket forceps (Fig. 8.5), the shaver or the cutter according to the site and nature of the area requiring excision. Around the patella, 90° angulated basket forceps (Fig. 8.6) are appropriate, because the direction of the instrument is tangential to the articular surface. For proliferative fibrillated lesions the shaver or the cutter is preferred (Fig. 8.7).

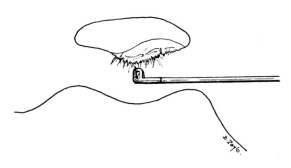

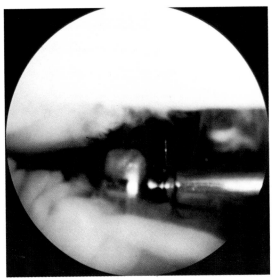

Figure 8.6. *Using the 90° angulated basket forceps for the patellar articular surface.*

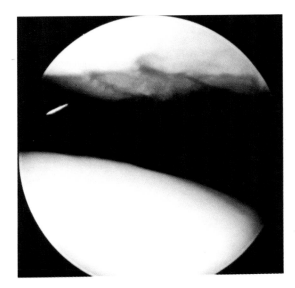

Figure 8.7. *Appearance of the residual patellar cartilage after arthroscopic shaving.*

If there is an indication for division of an associated lateral patellar retinaculum, this can be performed arthroscopically, although bleeding may be difficult to control.

Osteoarthrosis

The arthroscopic appearance corresponds to the bony involvement in relation to the cartilage involvement shown by radiographs which indicate condensation, osteophytes and geodes. *The cartilagenous involvement* is extensive both superficially and deep. In femorotibial osteoarthrosis (Fig. 8.8) only the anterior part may remain healthy; the knee must be fully flexed, thereby exposing the posterior part where lesions predominate, and where the subchondral bone is commonly exposed. Similar involvement is seen in the posterior part of the tibial plateau. In the patellofemoral compartment, it is more usually the lateral regions that are involved (Fig. 8.9). *The osseous involvement* is represented by increased density of the subchondral tissue, which appears whitish, eburnated and sometimes presents with longitudinal grooves which mate with similar lesions on the opposing articular surface. The presence and site of osteophytes depends on the type of arthrosis—thus, they may be seen on the borders of the patella or at the trochlear margin, peripherally around the tibial plateau, or on the sides of the femoral condyles. *Associated lesions* comprise involvement of the synovial membrane which may be hypertrophied and present with either an inflammatory or a sclerotic appearance; the menisci may present the usual appearance of meniscosis in tibiofemoral involvement. Occasionally, transverse rupture at the junctions of the posterior and middle thirds of the menisci may be seen (see Chapter 5). In some instances, complex lesions are seen comprising a diffuse softening and ragged appearance of the menisci with cleavages, fissures and tongues.

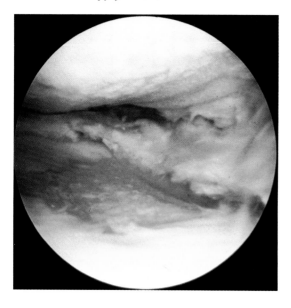

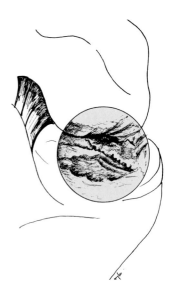

Figure 8.8. *Medial tibiofemoral arthrosis: the subchondral bone of the femur and tibia are visible with anteroposteriorly directed grooves. There remains a bed of cartilage in the anterior part of the femoral condyle and tibial plateau. There is an associated degenerative meniscosis.*

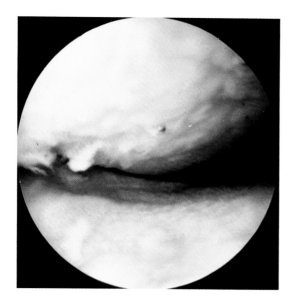

Figure 8.9. *Patellofemoral arthrosis.*

Arthroscopic management

Several possibilities exist:

Lavage may have a pain-relieving effect, although the value and duration of this is difficult to assess.

Synovial excision can be achieved by use of a shaver. It can be employed at sites of hypertrophy and inflammation either at femorotibial or at patellofemoral locations.

Meniscal excision is an appropriate here as for traumatic conditions. More than an excision, the procedure consists of a regularization which can be performed in a very economical fashion; thus a transverse rupture can be sufficiently excised, and other degenerative areas can be smoothed (using the cutter) retaining healthy meniscal tissue. It is always necessary to conserve a residual intact wall even though this may be very narrow; this continuity maintains to some extent the supportive role of the meniscus.

Excision of osteophytes is best achieved using a small reamer (Figs 8.10 and 8.11). The difficulty of the procedure can be significant in areas of limited access.

Cortical abrasion (Fig. 8.12) involves a superficial excision of the subchondral cortical bone of several millimetres thickness; it is not designed to expose spongy bone, but only to remove a superficial sclerosed avascular area of

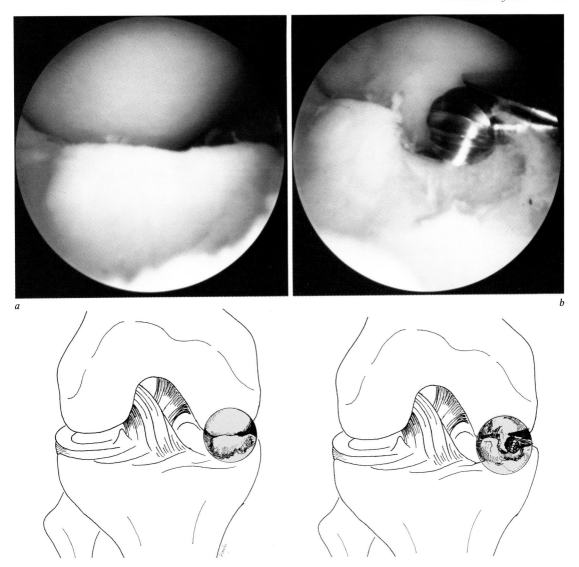

Figure 8.10. *Osteophyte. (a) Marginal anterior osteophyte of the medial tibial plateau; (b excision using a burr.*

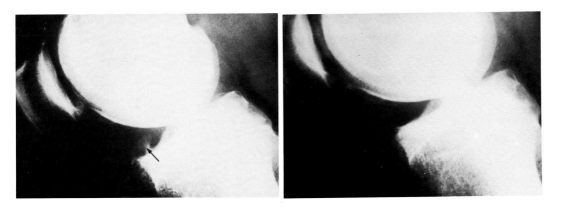

Figure 8.11. *Osteophyte (continued). Radiographic appearance before and after excision of a marginal anterior osteophyte of the medial tibial plateau.*

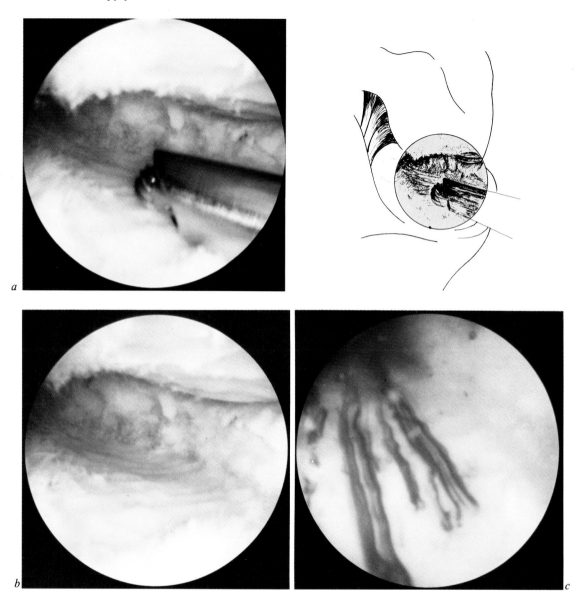

Figure 8.12. *Abrasion of the cortical bone of the medial tibiofemoral compartment. (a) This has been effected using a burr, raising one or two millimetres of the subchondral cortical bone; (b) the appearance of the femoral condyle and of the tibial plateau after osseous abrasion; (c) assessment of the adequacy of abrasion after release of the tourniquet as indicated by the bleeding.*

cortical bone, thereby allowing some degree of revascularization and the formation of neo-cartilage. Cortical abrasion can be performed only in areas entirely denuded of articular cartilage. The reamer operates in a transverse direction, beginning in the posterior part of the tibial condyle and progressively moving forwards. In the case of the patella, cortical abrasion is also applicable, but the tangential access necessary is more difficult. Following the

procedure in the literature a period of two months without weightbearing is necessary in order to allow the formation of sufficient neo-cartilage (Fig. 8.13).

In summary, diagnostic arthroscopy allows: assessment of the extent of the arthrosis (especially with respect to its depth and cartilagenous involvement); assessment of the state of the other articular compartment of, in

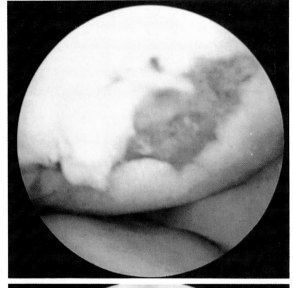

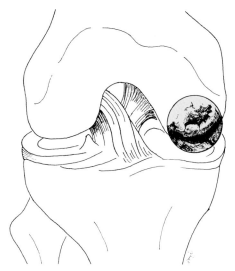

a

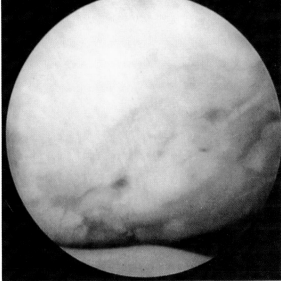

Figure 8.13. *Result of cortical abrasion of the medial femoral condyle. (a) Appearance before abrasion. There exists a mobile flap of cartilage. The subchondral cortex is visible. (b) Appearance three months after subchondral abrasion, showing total recovering with pseudocartilage.*

b

particular, the tibiofemoral joints, in order to judge the indications and likely results of osteotomy, and the evaluation of associated lesions, particularly of the menisci and the synovial membrane.

Operative arthroscopy must be viewed in a surgical context and does not offer a substitute when appropriate indications for osteotomy, for example, prevail. Indications are: the need for arthroscopic meniscectomy when, as is common in certain femorotibial arthroses, the symptomatology relates more to the mechanical effects of meniscal involvement; clinical

evaluation and radiology should accompany such procedures in order to detect the correct time for an osteotomy. Cortical abrasion associated with various acts on the menisci, the synovium, and osteophytes, is sometimes irksome because of the need for nonweight-bearing afterwards. The choice must be very selective, involving sufficient exposure of the subchondral bone and little or no angular deformity of the knee into valgus and varus. Sometimes, cortical abrasion offers the only alternative to the insertion of a prosthesis and may be preferable, especially in the young subject.

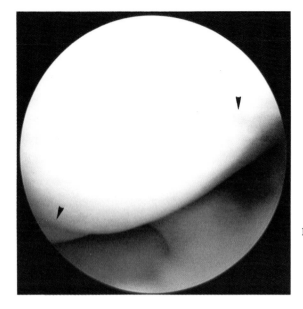

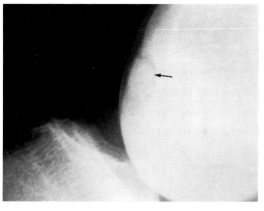

Figure 8.14. *Osteochondritis of the medial femoral condyle.*

Osteochondritis

The most common site is the medial femoral condyle and the arthroscopic appearances are variable. When the articular cartilage is intact, it may be difficult to localize the lesion. It is necessary to search carefully, guided by the radiographic localization, for a localized projection of the articular surface circumscribed by a furrow. Palpation using the arthroscopy hook may detect a softening of the whole zone (Fig. 8.14). At a later stage, the diagnosis is easy in that an osteocartilagenous sequestrum has developed and its site of detachment may be easily seen (Fig. 8.15). Once complete detachment has occurred, the sequestrum forms a foreign body, which may be more or less difficult to find; location may, of course, be helped by a pre-operative radiograph.

With regard to methods of treatment, we have no experience in the fixation of an osteochondral fragment under arthroscopic control, although we have removed a screw previously used for its fixation by an open procedure (Fig. 8.16). Our current treatment comprises removal of a sequestrum (when

large, it may be necessary to fragment it using a burr, morselizing forceps or disc forceps), the removal of any other foreign bodies from the joint, smoothing of the cartilagenous borders of the cavity using nibbling forceps, and the revitalization of the floor of the cavity using a burr, which seems to be more effective than the perforation recommended by Pridie (Fig. 8.17).

Areas of osteonecrosis can sometimes be treated similarly to osteochondritis (Fig. 8.18), but arthroscopic management alone is rarely indicated—often, osteotomy or a prosthesis are required; however, arthroscopy can usefully assess the potential, especially for osteotomy.

Osteochondral fracture

Arthroscopy allows precise evaluation of the fracture site and the recovery of loose bodies in the joint. Sometimes, in a case of traumatic haemarthrosis, the fracture area may be identified when it is not visible on radiographs; if the femoral condyle is involved, patellofemoral instability may also occur, introducing an additional ligamentous problem.

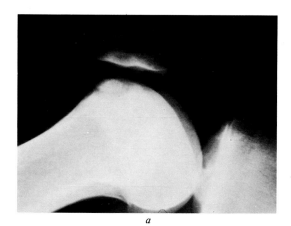

a

Figure 8.15. *Osteochondritis of the medial margin of the trochlear surface of the femur with sequestrum in process of separation. (a) Radiographic appearance; (b) arthroscopic appearance; (c) excision of the sequestra using disc forceps.*

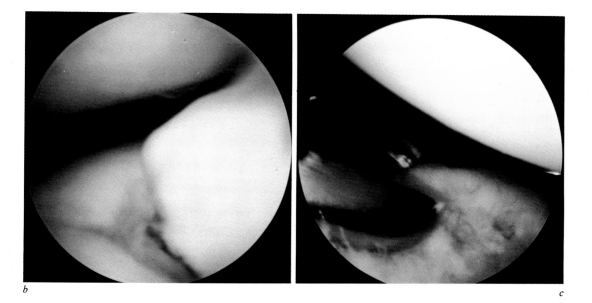

b

c

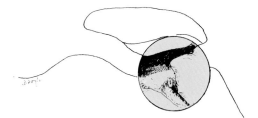

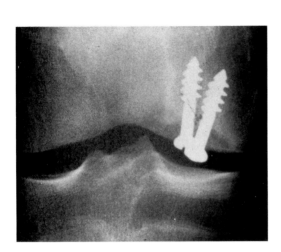

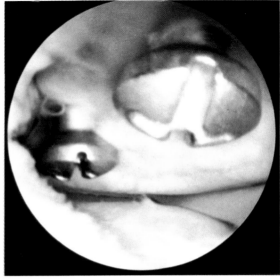

Figure 8.16. *Osteochondritis screwed. Prominence of the screw heads have eroded the articular surface of the tibial plateau. The screws were removed at arthroscopy.*

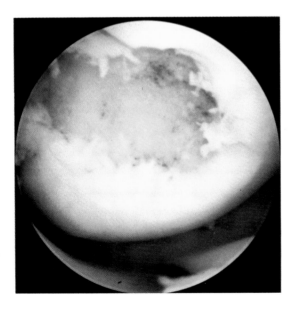

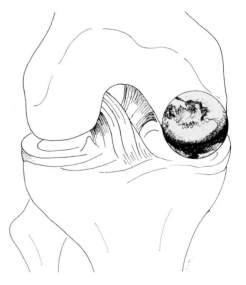

Figure 8.17. *Appearance of an osteochondritis niche after excision of the sequestrum and freshening by abrasion.*

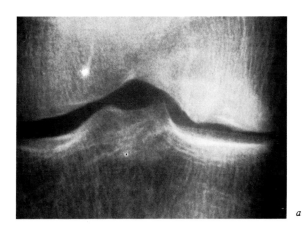

a

Figure 8.18. *Osteonecrosis of the medial femoral conyle. (a) Radiographic appearance; (b) the osteocartilagenous sequestrum; (c) abrasion using a burr; (d) appearance at close of procedure. The medial meniscus has also been smoothed.*

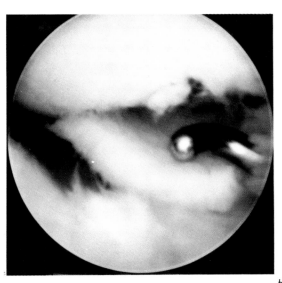

b

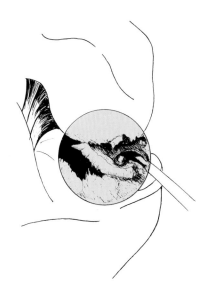

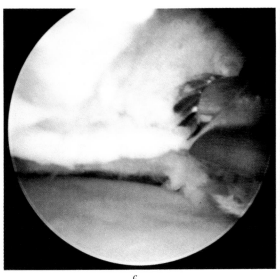

c

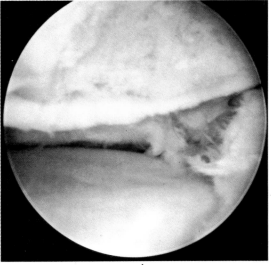

d

9

Foreign bodies

Arthroscopy is indicated for the discovery, removal and identification of the source of foreign bodies.

Clinical features and diagnosis

The clinical signs are usually characteristic, the patient describing episodes of transitory blocking, of pain, sensation of something moving in the joint, and of localized swelling. More rarely, it is possible to palpate a mobile hard mass, which may always reside in, or transitorily disappear from, a localized area. The radiograph will show radio-opaque foreign bodies. Sometimes the detected body is clinically silent. Careful study of successive radiographs will identify whether the foreign material is intra- or extra-articular, and whether it is mobile. Arthroscopy allows assessment of spurious, mistaken, or radio-transparent foreign bodies. Sometimes a foreign body may be an unexpected finding, although this is rare.

Sources of foreign bodies

Synovial (Figs 9.1 and 9.2): under the general heading of osteochondromatosis.

Chondral or osteochondral: due to *trauma* resulting from frequent episodes of patellar instability, which often detach a chondral or osteochondral fragment in some cases from the patella itself, or in others from the medial femoral condyle; *osteochondritis*, or *arthrosic degeneration*—in many cases the exact site of origin of the osteochondral fragment may not be found.

Meniscal: either from spontaneous detachments, or from lost fragments after surgery or arthroscopic work.

Extrinsic causes: for example, a parasite (filaria) or a piece of an operating instrument.

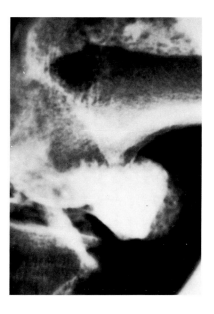

Figure 9.1. *Arthrography demonstrating the presence of chondromata, in particular seen in the posterior compartments.*

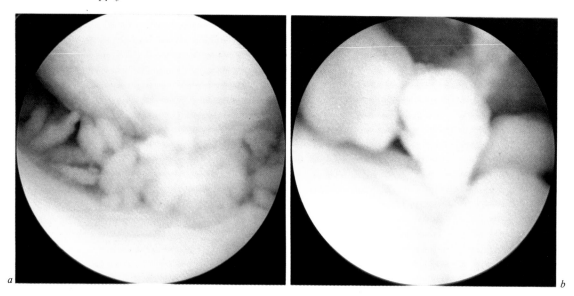

Figure 9.2. *(a) Numerous chondromata situated in the anteromedial compartment. (b) View as the chondromata are approached.*

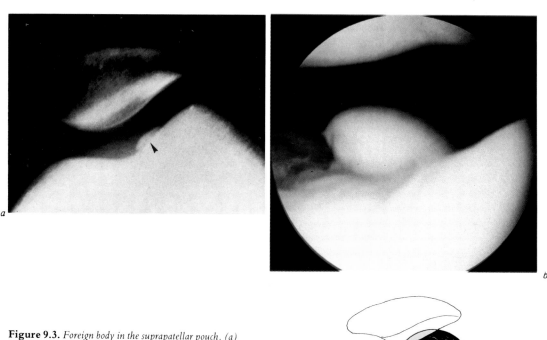

Figure 9.3. *Foreign body in the suprapatellar pouch. (a) Radiograph; (b) arthroscopic appearance.*

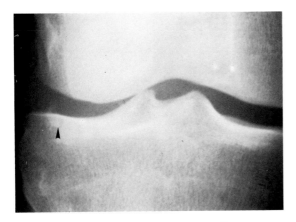

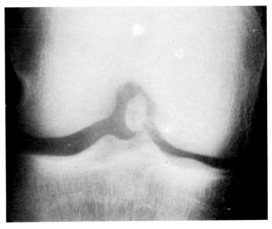

Figure 9.4. *Foreign body under the anterior horn of the lateral meniscus.*

a

The site of foreign bodies

In about 50 per cent of cases, the object locates in the suprapatellar pouch (Fig. 9.3), which explains the need for adequate distension in order to obtain as clear a vision as possible. In other instances, the foreign body is equally likely to reside in the anterior, posterior, or collateral recesses of the joint. The risk of not finding a foreign body exists especially at certain sites, notably in the area near the popliteal hiatus, or under the anterior or posterior horn of the lateral meniscus (Fig. 9.4). A synovial proliferation in the intercondylar area can hide a loose body (Fig. 9.5).

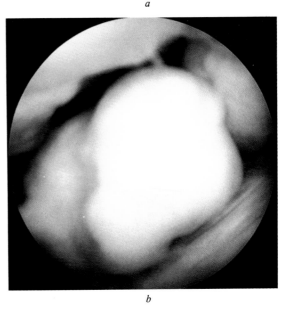

b

Figure 9.5. *Foreign body in the intercondylar notch. (a) Radiograph; (b) arthroscopic appearance.*

Types of foreign body

These can be free and very mobile, especially when not large, and when spherical. When oblong and polished, they may be difficult to grasp. Occasionally, the foreign body is not free, but retains a synovial pedicle and floats in the joint cavity; these examples may cause intermittent locking always manifesting the same character, because the foreign body remains located in the same area. Finally, they may become impacted in proliferated synovial tissue and become immobilized, sometimes not producing mechanical symptoms. An osteochondritis fragment in the process of

sequestrating and separating may be regarded as an intermediate form of loose body formation.

The size varies from a few millimetres to several centimetres and exceptionally, the volume is so great that morselization must be effected before extraction is possible, even after having considerably enlarged the port of exit. The number can also vary, ranging from a single one to some hundreds in the case of osteochondromatosis. Consistency depends on the nature of the foreign body, whether chondral, osteochondral or fibrous; occasionally fragments of menisci might be present.

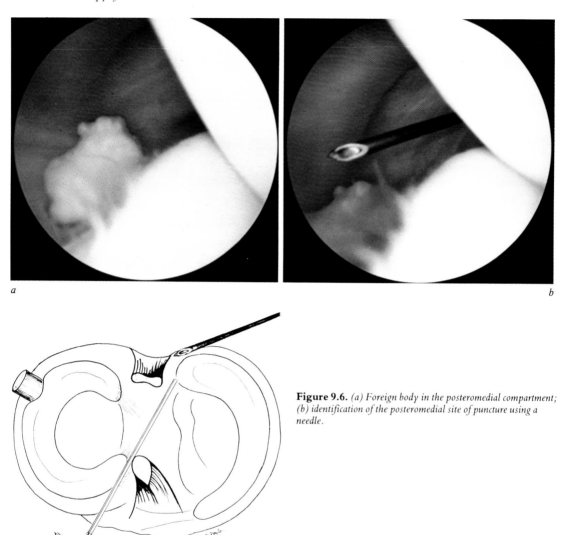

a   *b*

Figure 9.6. *(a) Foreign body in the posteromedial compartment; (b) identification of the posteromedial site of puncture using a needle.*

Technique for removal

The limb should be set up as for routine arthroscopy, ensuring that the posterior medial and lateral compartments are accessible. Atypical ports of entry are sometimes required.

Identification of the site (Figs 9.6 and 9.7) is easy if the loose body is palpable in the suprapatellar pouch or in the collateral recesses, in which case the knee should be held in one position in order to avoid the matter escaping elsewhere. Sometimes, an immediate pre-operative radiograph is useful to identify the current situation but, in most cases, a full systematic exploration is necessary. It is useful to stop the irrigation flow in order to prevent the foreign body from continuously skating around inside the joint cavity. Digital pressure locally over all areas of the knee may cause the fragment to appear, especially when it has become lodged in some place of difficult access.

The search begins in the suprapatellar pouch and afterwards is extended first down the medial collateral recess and then down the

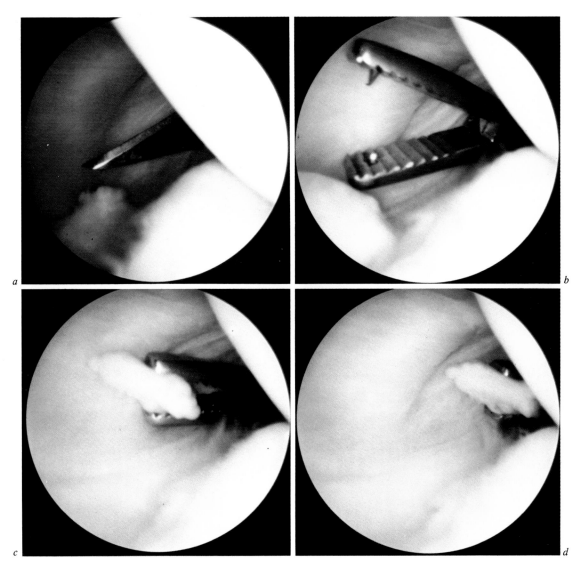

Figure 9.7. *Foreign body in the posteromedial compartment (continued). (a) Puncture with the knife; (b), (c,d) grasping the foreign body and its extraction.*

lateral collateral recess. If no foreign body is found in these areas, the intercondylar notch should be crossed into the posteromedial and posterolateral compartments.

Once discovered, the foreign body should be trapped and placed in an area of easy access in order to remove it while maintaining immobility. Immobility can be achieved by stopping the turbulence created by the lavage system, by digital pressure, with the aid of a transcutaneous needle, or by application of the arthroscopy hook.

A sufficiently large port of direct approach facilitates extraction. The size of the incision must reflect the size of the body to be removed. Sometimes, a more accurate appraisal of the size can be gained by palpation with the hook, rather than by using the arthroscope, which causes magnification. The grasp on the foreign body must be secure. If it is of elongated form, a hold on one of its ends is preferable, so that it can be extracted in the direction of its axis. Several types of forceps can be used: Kocher, meniscus forceps or disc forceps.

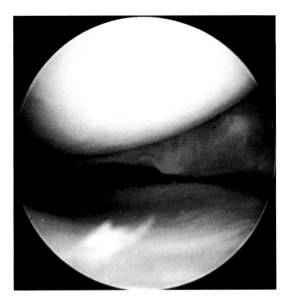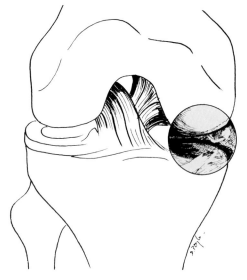

Figure 9.8. *Abnormally short meniscus must lead to a search for a meniscal fragment.*

When very numerous foreign bodies are present, as in osteochondromatosis, a lavage technique is simple and more effective than an individual approach. At the anteromedial aspect, a large evacuation port can be established and a rapid circulation of lavage fluid can then wash out all the fragments. The cannula should be placed systematically into superior, anterior and posterior compartments successively.

When the foreign body is pedunculated or embedded, a preliminary dissection may be necessary before extraction is possible. Before dividing a pedicle, it is always better to grasp the foreign body in some way so that it is not lost.

In the cases of certain soft and large foreign masses, it may be necessary to morselize them and then to extract them by aspiration. The disc forceps or the burr may be necessary in order to reduce hard, large bodies to manageable size. Motorized instruments (cutter or shaver) have the advantage of aspirating small fragments made at the same time as cutting.

Identification of site of origin

This must be performed systematically with regard to the radiographic appearance. The discovery of a foreign body must *always* arouse the suspicion of a source which could be the cause of future troubles. Conversely, for example, a narrow meniscus, even when regular in outline, should lead the operator to search for a meniscal fragment (Fig. 9.8).

Escape of a foreign body

There is nothing more irritating than losing a foreign body after having seen or even grasped it, and to have to spend many minutes trying to relocate it. In cases of difficulty, there should be no hesitation in starting the exploration all over again as detailed above. Two possibilities should be borne in mind however: the foreign body may have been ejected during the lavage and may be in the bucket, or it may have passed out of the knee cavity but become impacted in the subcutaneous tissue. This can occur if the skin incision is not sufficiently large to allow its removal; due to the local distension of the subcutaneous tissue, a fairly small fragment may be very difficult to locate.

While removal of foreign bodies appears very simple in principle, this is not always the case. Sometimes, such arthroscopies can take the longest!

10

Complications of arthroscopy

As in all surgical procedures, arthroscopy is not without complication. While rare, the knowledge of such complications is a guide to prevention as well as management.

Intra-operative complications

1. Anaesthesia

There are no complications specific to anaesthesia for arthroscopy, whether general or local.

2. Articular surface damage

Iatrogenic lesions of the articular cartilage are difficult to evaluate with respect to frequency and severity. They are more likely to occur in those knees which are tight, or in which the ports of entry have not been appropriately selected. The commonest instruments producing injury are the knife, the trocar, the telescope of the arthroscope, or other operative instruments.

To avoid these articular cartilage lesions, it is always necessary to ensure an optimal visual access, and instruments should never be introduced forcefully. Always manipulate the knee carefully when there is an instrument *in situ* and never hesitate to change a port of entry if this would facilitate the work.

3. Ligament and tendon injury

The medial collateral ligament can be easily damaged by excessive valgus force. This is commoner in patients of more than forty years of age and in whom the knee is difficult to open on the medial side. The greatest care should be taken in cases where there already exists a fresh sprain of the medial collateral ligament, since excessive valgus force risks completing this. It is suspected that in some cases valgus stressing has been responsible for the inflammatory response of the medial collateral ligament and for prolonged post-operative pain.

Iatrogenic lesions of the *anterior cruciate ligament* are very exceptional. More frequent, is a lesion of the *popliteal tendon*. Lateral meniscectomy is sometimes difficult and forceps can damage the popliteal tendon whilst opening the popliteal hiatus. It is absolutely essential to locate the popliteal tendon during peripheral resection in this difficult area by exerting traction on the residual meniscal fragment before cutting and, because the popliteal tendon is relatively fixed, this allows selective section of the meniscus without cutting the tendon.

4. Meniscal

During anteromedial incision, the medial meniscus can be cut. In order to avoid this, introduction of a needle under visual control is most useful.

5. Vascular

A lace-like venous plexus exists over the anteromedial port area and its transillumination enables visualization so that incision can be conducted a little distant from them.

Synovectomy can be accompanied by significant haemorrhage, especially in such conditions as villonodular synovitis. Abundant lavage after the tourniquet is let down is helpful, when one should ensure that the evacuated fluid becomes progressively clear.

Damage to the popliteal artery is fortunately very rare.

6. Instrument breakage

This is likely to occur more frequently when the operator is inexperienced, but always remains a possibility. The instruments most likely to break include the scissors and the basket forceps, but any instrument can fracture, even the hook, the burr or the blades. In order to avoid such fracture, always use the most appropriate instrument. Never force an instrument; always ensure that instruments are well cared for (note that sharpening can sometimes lead to fatigue and fracture), and while the checking of instruments on the table is the duty of the assistant, their visualization inside the joint is often revealing because of the magnification effect of the arthroscope. Any instrument which is not functioning properly may be the source of a *future* breakage and should be changed.

The recovery of broken material is possible using the arthroscope, and some devices can facilitate such removal. In particular, a magnet can be slid into the joint to attract a metallic fragment otherwise difficult to retrieve. Frequently, fragments slip into the posterior compartments, hence the usefulness of posterior approaches.

Post-operative complications

Vascular

Distension or compression can cause a late vascular complication, in particular, post-operative swelling of the leg, or rupture of a popliteal cyst, both of which are usually corrected within a few days. Certain precautions prevent such complications; notably knowledge of the pre-operative circulatory state or of the presence of a popliteal cyst, and the use of a lavage system of reasonable pressure and a correct evacuation method.

Phlebitis is not rare despite the limited duration of the operation and early post-operative mobilization. Pre-anaesthetic assessment may detect risk factors, when anticoagulant therapy may be advisable.

Post-operative swelling in the region of the arthroscopy port may be haemorrhagic or serous. Usually, the volume is small and requires no particular systematic treatment. Local application of ice for three quarters of an hour, three or four times a day, is advised and the first application should be made as soon as possible post-operatively. Compressive dressing is also useful.

Occasionally, a severe swelling may demand aspiration and if the collection is haemorrhagic, a low grade pyrexia may be noted after evacuation. Swelling of this type settles spontaneously within a few days, but sometimes takes two to three weeks.

Certain circumstances predispose to post-arthroscopic swelling. Immediate post-operative swelling is likely in patients who presented with pre-operative swelling and in whom symptoms have lasted for a long time; after arthroscopic synovectomy or division of a plica; after complete meniscal resection, particularly of the lateral side, or after severe sprains.

Chronic persistent swelling occurs in certain typical cases of a knee with advanced arthrosis or chondrocalcinosis, rheumatoid synovitis, degenerate lateral meniscus conditions, amyotropia of the quadriceps muscle and 'insufficient arthroscopic treatment' (see 'Late complications' below). Treatment of chronic hydrarthrosis relates to its cause; for example, building up the quadriceps musculature in cases of amyotrophy is important.

In certain examples, the intra-articular injection of hydrocortisone may settle the formation of hydrarthrosis.

Neurological

Such complications are rare. If the precautions described earlier are observed there should be no risk of damage to the lateral popliteal nerve during posterolateral puncture of the knee. Compression syndromes affecting the medial or lateral popliteal nerves can occur in the presence of large popliteal cysts or as a result of the prolonged use of a tourniquet. Usually, compression lesions are reversible, but with a variable delay. Careful restriction of the duration of use of a tourniquet is without doubt a major preventative element.

More frequently, the sensory nerves are involved, particularly of the internal saphenous nerve. This may affect the small terminal branches, and recuperation may take a long time or even remain incomplete.

Muscular

Various types are frequent. *Muscle pains* may arise as a result of pressure from the tourniquet or the stirrup but usually they regress spontaneously. The point of puncture through the superomedial port can remain abnormally painful if the direction of the cannula for admission of fluid has not been directed towards the suprapatellar pouch.

Wasting of the musculature is also frequent, perhaps related to the pre-operative condition or secondary to the arthroscopy itself. Electromyographic studies have been made which suggest that the use of a tourniquet can precipitate electrical changes over several months. Similarly, the presence of an effusion can cause reflex muscle wasting. The two factors, tourniquet and arthrosis, contribute to the quadriceps muscle wasting, the significance of which is well known.

Muscle atrophy is usually prevented by an early return to normal activities, but this is not always the case. In general, a few sessions of routine physiotherapy are valuable, with static quadriceps exercises of increasing vigour and, later, more strenuous measures, especially for patients participating in sports.

Cutaneous

Although not serious, some cutaneous complications are frequent. Reactions to skin disinfectants, allergies, and haematoma due to over forceful pressure against the arthroscopy stirrup can all occur.

Skin closure may be performed with sutures or steristrips, while some arthroscopists do not close the skin but only apply a sterile dressing.

Local subcutaneous inflammation merits close attention because of the proximity of the underlying joint. Usually, such infections are successfully treated locally.

Synovial cyst formation is frequent, but usually resolves spontaneously within one to two months, during which period they may cause discomfort.

Aseptic fistula formation is rare. It is likely to be precipitated by an effusion followed by a too vigorous attempt to flex the knee, which creates high pressure inside the joint. Aspiration of fluid followed by a restricted flexion exercise programme is usually sufficient for cure. Occasionally, it is necessary to insert a deep stitch in order to close the fistula.

Cutaneous necrosis is possible. This usually relates to the use of local anaesthetics including lignocaine and adrenaline.

Infection

This is rare. According to the literature, it occurs in about 1:2500 arthroscopy procedures. Overwhelmingly, the causative organism is *Staphylococcus aureus*. The incidence has proved commoner in combined arthroscopy and subsequent surgery, even though the latter may have been extra-articular.

It is treated in the same way as ordinary septic arthritis.

With regard to prevention, care should be taken with the sterilization of instruments bearing in mind their repeated use, meticulous attention to the condition of the skin pre-operatively (the short incisions in arthroscopy must not be regarded as immune to the risk of infection), and extra care when arthroscopy and surgery are combined—change of instruments, of blades, etc.

Algodystrophy

Although arthroscopy may be regarded as minor surgery, algodystrophy can occur. The prognosis and development of such a condition is similar to that from any other cause.

Late complications

Failure of an arthroscopic treatment may be regarded as a late complication, although such failure is not frequent and usually relates to an insufficient therapeutic procedure during the first arthroscopy: for example, horizontal lesions of the menisci and meniscal cysts. Foreign bodies may have been incompletely removed, or the arthroscopic treatment was not appropriate for the pathological condition found at the first arthroscopy.

Pathological conditions can evolve secondarily: for example, osteochondromatosis, the redevelopment of a plica, and secondary aggravation of a chondropathy.

Finally, it should be mentioned that articular cartilage complications are no different from those encountered after conventional meniscal surgery, and terminal loss of range of flexion may make crouching difficult.

11

Pitfalls and failures in arthroscopy

It is useful to summarize these, although many have been mentioned earlier.

Optical and video apparatus

The success of all arthroscopic procedures depends upon the quality of the optical system.

1. Natural wear and tear

The lighting system

Lamps have a limited life and their quality of light naturally deteriorates with time. It is necessary to know how to change a lamp, but beware of severe burns. The cold light cable also has a limited life. The principle cause of deterioration, even with proper routine care, occurs during repeated sterilizations and the microtraumata due to folding of the cable.

The camera

Deterioration is inevitable with time. This is variable according to type, but is especially marked in cameras with television tubes. Repeated washing and cleaning accelerates aging of the optical elements. However careful the arthroscopist may be, this deterioration will result in progressive diminution in quality of light-transmission. For this reason, it is always wise to choose a light source of sufficient power and a sensitive camera.

2a. Avoidable wear and tear: mechanical damage

Minor repeated damage. Much of this is preventable. The arthroscope is very sensitive to shock either from something inside the joint or from another instrument. It is always necessary to be careful to avoid contact with a cutter, a shaver or a burr which, owing to vibration, can severely damage the optical system. A motorized instrument must be kept at a distance; if it is a cutter or a shaver, the port of entry should be on the side opposite to that through which the arthroscope has been inserted, in order to protect the optical end of the arthroscope; the sheath should completely enclose the telescope and it should slightly exceed the length of the optical system, thereby protecting it. Penetration of the synovial membrane must be performed without using the optical system *in situ*, to avoid damage not only to the articular surface, but also to the telescope itself.

Torsional stresses are very traumatic for the cold light source cable. The arthroscope telescope is protected from twisting by the sleeve, but this can be overcome. With regard to the cold light cable itself, folding is unavoidable to some extent, but sharp angles must be avoided, otherwise the optical fibres deteriorate particularly rapidly. A simple rubber sleeve will prevent excessive folding, allowing at the same time disinfection in the fluid bath.

The cable which joins the camera to the light source is also fragile and can deteriorate if one allows torsion or acute folding to take place.

Serious mechanical accidents such as dropping the instruments, especially the camera, are unpardonable with such expensive equipment. Direct contact of the cutting elements of the shaver or of the cutter against the arthroscope is very dangerous, especially inside the joint.

2b. Avoidable wear and tear: sterilizing solutions

Sterilizing agents together with salinity will eventually have a corrosive effect on the camera and the lighting cable. Application of the rinsing fluids should be continued for no longer than is necessary for the sterilizing effect to be achieved.

Defects in construction can always result in an early deterioration of instrument. It is not superfluous to have a second arthroscope always at hand in case of failure.

3. Poor functioning of the optical and visual equipment

Abnormal colour with red or yellow or blue predominance suggests that the camera is poorly adjusted to the colour temperature of the light source.

A foggy image deteriorating during the course of the arthroscopy is a classic annoyance and may be due to humidity at the camera–arthroscope junction. Very careful drying here is essential.

A dim image indicates a defect in the light cable, in the light source itself, or perhaps in the telescope. Sometimes the voltage supply to the light source is insufficient.

A defective monitor image may relate simply to incorrect regulation of the receiver itself or, of particular annoyance, can be caused by electrical apparatus in the same or an adjacent operating theatre.

4. Breakdowns

Where the failure occurs at the outset or during the procedure, so that there is no longer an image on the monitor, two sources should be investigated: failure of transmission of the light and/or failure of transmission of the image. In order to save time, especially tourniquet time,

it is necessary to have a check list. Methodically, the following points should be eliminated:

(a) Verification of the light source

• Inspect the telescope for fracture of the terminal lens and check vision directly through it by examination of a light source; verify the quality of the zone of reception of the light on the arthroscope.
• Check that the light source cable junction is correctly screwed together.
• Ensure that light is being transmitted by the cable, that its ferrule is properly inserted and not defective. When the end of a lighted cable is inspected, the quality of conduction can be verified and if there exist numerous dark areas, this suggests multiple fractures of the fibre optic system. If too numerous, these will seriously reduce the quality of transmission.
• Check the lamp, the fuses, and the electrical supply.

(b) Checking the camera and the monitor

• Check the electrical supply and function of the amplifier.

Operating instruments

Arthroscopic instruments are necessarily of good quality, precise, and appropriate for intra-articular manipulation. They are used repetitively and deterioration to the point of fracture is inevitable.

(a) Deterioration of instruments

There are various causes:

Mechanical torsion occurs mainly with the basket forceps, the scissors and the hook. A badly chosen port of approach is often responsible for unnecessary force, as, for example, during meniscectomy, where an instrument is bent around the femoral condyle.

Inappropriate use is exemplified by the use of basket forceps to remove osteophytes, whereas normally they are used for synovial membrane or for meniscal section.

Poor instrument maintenance. Slicing instruments such as basket forceps scissors lose their quality unless regularly sharpened. The operator risks forcing and therefore damaging them if they are too blunt. The same applies to motorized blades.

Failure of power instruments

● Failure of aspiration—debris can block the aspirating system; this can be easily checked and corrected.
● Failure of mechanical action is normally due to failure of a battery supply. Careful charging of batteries is always essential. Sometimes it is a loose connection (eg a pedal control) which causes failure.

It is always necessary to emphasize to staff the need for the most assiduous attention to arthroscopic apparatus, checking that meniscal, cartilagenous or synovial debris are removed.

(b) Instrument fracture

The hook, basket forceps, the knife and the scissors are especially prone to this type of misadventure. Most frequently a component such as the jaw of the basket forceps or the blade of the scissors breaks off. Several precautions should be observed to avoid this type of accident: a careful check first by the assistant, and then while the instrument is magnified inside the joint, should be routine; the careful use of the instrument itself, avoiding undue force, is important, and always ensure that cutting devices are sharp.

Technical failure

Failure may be due to bad visual access or inability to perform surgery inside the confines of the joint.

Causes of a defective image

(i.) The arthroscope may be extra-articular.

(ii.) Some fragment of tissue like meniscus, cartilage, or a synovial fringe is interposed.

In the latter case, lavage performed retrograde through the arthroscope can sometimes clear the offending debris.

Sometimes fibrils or shavings of articular cartilage may impede direct vision. These can be removed using either basket forceps or a motorized instrument.

(iii.) Poor irrigation. This may be due to a malsited or too small an admission cannula; insufficient pressure; bags of lavage fluid being too low, or poor circulation of the fluid from the suprapatellar pouch in relation to valgus and varus stressing or flexion. In order to avoid this last problem, the knee should be relaxed periodically so as to allow a free circulation.

The evacuation of the lavage fluid may be insufficient. This may be due to the outlet being too narrow or tortuous, inhibiting flow. Occasionally, one has forgotten to open taps situated in the sheath of the arthroscope. Two commonly obvious but overlooked sources of annoyance are an empty irrigation source, and the cutting off of the supply by kinking the tube in some way.

Adequate irrigation is particularly important in cases of joint effusion, haemarthrosis, or after arthrography, when it is necessary to evacuate tiresome opaque liquid in order to obtain adequate vision. If the fluid becomes obscured by blood, this can be due to several causes including partial deflation of the tourniquet which then acts as a venous obstruction only.

Again, excessive aspiration near the site of operation can encourage bleeding. From time to time it is useful to clamp off the aspiration side of the lavage system.

When using motorized equipment, it is necessary to clamp off the exit of fluid from the arthroscope sheath. Without this precaution, bubbles will form and disturb vision.

Finally, it should be noted that bullae or collapse of the synovial membrane can be brought about by excessive aspiration if the irrigating source is inadequate. The two should be harmonized in order to maintain optimal filling, especially when using motorized equipment which also aspirates.

Conclusion

Arthroscopy utilizes sophisticated apparatus designed for the production of intra-articular images and for endoscopic surgery. The operator must know the different causes of instrument failure if he is to avoid disappointment and to make the learning process easier. Accordingly, it is wise to seek preventive measures, and to be prepared for possible accidents. Prevention is better than cure.

12

Information for the patient

It seems to us highly desirable to give the patient some information about the arthroscopic procedure which he is to undergo. These explanations concerning the state of his knee should be made at the time of consultation, and may be made much simpler if a model is used (Fig. 12.1). We recommend the use of systematic documentation which will avoid errors of omission.

Arthroscopy of the knees (a document given to the patient)

The aim of arthroscopy of the knee is to see inside the joint either to make a diagnosis of what is wrong or, sometimes, to perform some surgical work inside without actually making a big incision.

1. Technique

Arthroscopy is done in the operating theatre under general or local anaesthetic. The arthroscope is a tube several millimetres in diameter which has an optical system and a lighting system. It is coupled to a micro video camera so that what is happening can be seen on a television screen and recorded on a tape recorder if necessary.

The arthroscope is put into the knee through a very small incision, or sometimes several

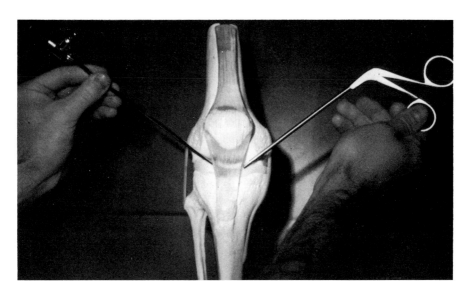

Figure 12.1. *A model of the knee facilitates the explanation to the patient of the pathology and of the arthroscopic procedure.*

small incisions, because it may be necessary also to insert fine instruments. During the investigation the knee is inflated with special liquid.

2. The indications for arthroscopy

(a) Diagnosis

Arthroscopy can be used to find out exactly what is causing trouble inside the knee, whether it be pain, swelling, locking, or feelings of instability. In the majority of cases, clinical and radiological examinations have already provided an approximate diagnosis and arthroscopy is indicated only if the information is insufficient.

Arthroscopy allows examination of the whole of the inside of the joint, the state of the lining or synovial membrane, the state of the articular cartilage of the knee cap, the femur or the tibia, the state of the menisci and of the central crossed ligaments.

(b) Operative arthroscopy

A certain number of operations can be performed through the arthroscope without necessarily opening the knee. This has been made possible by special miniaturized instruments having a high degree of precision.

The operation can be conducted, with respect to the synovial lining of the joint, by excision of adhesions and of replicated folds; the menisci can be removed totally or partially, according to the degree of damage, but it is always possible to conserve the healthy part when the operation is performed through an arthroscope; the surface of the bone, the articular cartilage, can be smoothed if it is grooved or irregular, or has lumps projecting into the joint. This smoothing can also be extended to the underlying bone if necessary. Finally, arthroscopy allows removal of small bony fragments or pieces of cartilage which escape into the joint, so-called foreign bodies.

3. Practical instructions

1. In the days preceding an arthroscopy operation and possible arthroscopic surgery, make sure that the doctor knows about any recent symptoms however trivial, such as rheumatism, pain in the chest etc., and above all if you have a temperature, even of moderate degree, because this may necessitate postponement of your operation.

All pre-operative preparation will be performed at the time of your admission. Do not attempt to shave or remove any hair around the knee which is to be treated. On arrival, tell the nurse if you have any sensitivity or allergy to depilatory creams.

2. Do not forget to bring any x-rays that you may possess.

3. On arrival at the hospital, tell the nurse of any skin disorders that you may have. However minor these may appear to be, it may be wiser to postpone your operation.

4. On the day of the operation you must fast so that you can be given an anaesthetic. So do not eat or drink anything without the agreement of the nurse who receives you.

You will be taken into the operating theatre and anaesthesia will be started after you have been put on the operating table. In the interests of hygiene do not talk in the operating theatre.

5. After waking up, do not attempt to get up and walk without the assistance of a nurse, because you may be a little giddy as a result of having had an anaesthetic.

6. You will be discharged from the clinic on the day after the arthroscopy. Occasionally, if you experience more discomfort than expected, or have a fever, you may need to remain in hospital for several days.

7. With regard to post-operative care of your knee after arthroscopy, during the first week do not attempt to bend the knee through more than 90°. You will be able to walk, sit, and climb stairs within a few days. Avoid standing for long periods. It is best to have periods lying down or seated, keeping your knee fully straightened and supported on a stool.

It is advisable to cool your knee four or five times a day by placing a plastic bag containing ice on it for about half an hour. If the cold is uncomfortable, you can put a piece of cloth between the plastic bag and your skin.

Practise contracting the front muscles of your thigh (the quadriceps) maintaining tension for some ten seconds at a time several times a day. Lift your leg as high as possible.

Do not attempt any sport without medical authorization.

8. The little incisions made by the surgeon will be closed by a stitch or a fine adhesive strip and covered by an adhesive dressing. Within a week, the dressing should be removed so as to expose the little scar to the air. Do not take a bath until the tenth post-operative day.

9. If you have an arthroscopic operation, you will come to see your surgeon again about one week after the operation. The surgeon may advise you to have some physiotherapy.

10. In common with all surgical operations, occasionally a complication can occur. Some bleeding can occur under the skin, inflammation can develop, a local infection may occur. Never hesitate to telephone if you have any worries, especially if you have excessive pain or cramp, a temperature above 38° Celsius, or a swelling of the knee. Moderate swelling is common, with a splashing sensation in the joint due to some of the liquid used during the arthroscopy remaining inside.

Bibliography

Arlet J, 'Essai de définition et de classification des arthroses,' *Séminaire annuel de rhumatologie, Clermont-Ferrand*, 24–25 November 1983.

Barrie HJ, 'The pathogenesis and significance of meniscal cysts', *J Bone Joint Surg* [Br.] (1979) **61**: 184–189.

Boyer Th, 'Lésions méniscales dégéneratives', *Séminaire d'arthroscopie. Palais des Congrès, Paris*, 25–27 April 1984.

Chassaing V, Parier J, Artigala Ph, 'L'arthroscopie opératoire dans le traitement, du kyste du ménisque externe. Technique. Résultats', *Journée de la Société Française d'Arthroscopie.* 15 December 1984, Versailles.

Chassaing V, Parier J, 'Désinsertion du segment postérieur du ménisque interne et externe. Problèmes diagnostiques et thérapeutiques en arthroscopie', *J de Med Lyon*, no. 1386, 11–15, February 1984.

Delee JC, Dickaut SC 'The discoid lateral-meniscus syndrome', *J Bone Joint Surg* (1982) **64A** (no. 7): 1068, September.

Dorfmann H, Dreyfus P, Justin-Besançon L, Sèze S (de), 'Arthroscopie du genou. État actuel de la question', *Sem Hôp Paris* (1970) **46** (no. 52): 3442–3450.

Ficat RP, *Cartilage et arthrose. Exploration fonctionnelle pathologique et thérapeutique* (Masson, 1979).

Hurter E, 'L'arthroscopie, nouvelle méthode d'exploration du genou', *Rev Chir Orthop* (1955) **41** (no. 5–6): 763–766.

Jackson RW, Dandy DJ, *Arthroscopy of the knee* (Grune and Stratton. Saint-Louis, 1977).

Johnson LL, *Diagnostic and surgical arthroscopy* (Second edition. The C.V. Mosby Company. Saint-Louis, Toronto, London, 1981).

Lemaire M, Combelles F, Miremad C, Van vooren P, 'Les désinsertions ménisco-capsulaires postéro-internes asso-ciées aux instabilités chroniques du genou par rupture du ligament croisé antérieur', *Rev Chir Orthop* (1984) **70** (no. 8): 613–622.

Miremad C, 'Radiological diagnosis and operative indications in posteromedial meniscocapsular lesions of the meniscus associated with rupture of the ACL'. *Third congress of the International Society of the knee.* Gleneagles, Scotland, 27 April–2 May 1983.

Mulhollan JS, Complications, AAOS Course, San Francisco, June 1980.

O'Connor RL, *O'Connor's textbook of arthroscopic surgery* (Ed. Heshmat Shahriaree. JB Lippincott. Philadelphia, 1984).

Patel D, 'Arthroscopie du genou. L'abord supéro-externe', *2es journées d'arthroscopie du genou*, 16–17 September 1983, Lyon.

Pellaci F, *Arthroscopia diagnostica* (Aulo Gaggi Editore. Bologna, 1983).

Saillant G, Benazet JP, Roy-Camille R 'Complications de l'arthroscopie', *2 journées d'arthroscopie du genou.* 16–17 September 1983, Lyon.

Seedhom B, 'Load bearing function of the meniscus; intact, torn, and meniscus after removal of a bucket handle tear', *Third congress of the International Society of the Knee. Gleneagles, Scotland*, 27 April–2 May 1983.

Tesson MC, Aignan M, Delbarre F, 'L'arthroscopie du genou. Technique, indications, résultats', *Presse Med* (1970) **78**: 2467–2471.

Trillat A, 'Lésions traumatiques du ménisque interne du genou. Classement anatomique et diagnostic clinique', *Rev Chir Orthop* (1962) **48**, (no. 5): 551–560.

Watanabe M, Ikeuchi H, 'L'arthroscopie'. *Encycl Med Chir Paris Appareil locomoteur.* 14 001 P-10 4-1981.

Index

Page numbers in *italic* refer to the illustrations

Arthroscopy of the Knee